PALEO DIET FOR WOMEN

120+ Recipes to Discover the Secrets of Rapid Weight Loss and A Healthy Lifestyle Using the Paleo Diet! All Low-carb and Ketogenic Recipes!

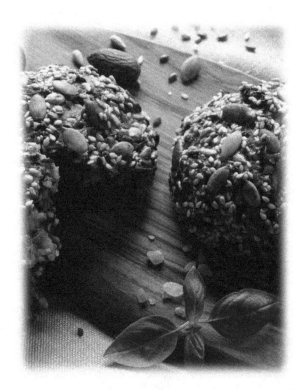

By

Robert Baker

TABLE OF CONTENT

INTRODUCTION

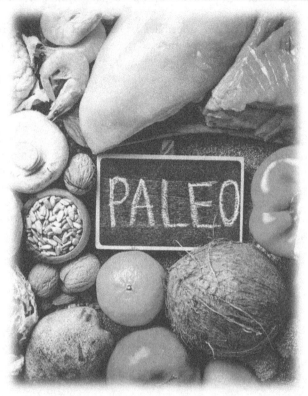

It's an epidemic in this country: people are overweight, tired, and eating poorly. The American diet is full of carbs, sugars, and processed foods that make us fat, feel malnourished, and too tired to do anything with our lives.

If you picked up this book, you're looking for a change. She's looking for a way to eat healthier and feel better. She also wants to lose weight. She realizes that the current Western diet is not working for her. Well, this book has the answer she's looking for.

Eat like a cave dweller! People refer to the paleo diet as the caveman diet because it is based on how humans ate over 10,000 years ago, before the advent of agriculture. People ate what was available through hunting and foraging, namely meat, fruits, vegetables, and nuts. Dairy products, carbohydrates, and anything else that was processed was not available to them.

Eating like a cave dweller has many benefits, the biggest of which is that they will be healthier and lose weight. It may take some dedication to give up the foods he is used to, but the results are more than worth it. Imagine being at a healthy weight for your body, having the energy to do all the activities you dream of, and feeling lean and mean, like the caveman of old.

He can lose weight. He can eat healthily. He can take control of his life. By eating the paleo diet, he will have all of these things.

THE BENEFITS OF THE PALEO DIET FOR WOMEN

The paleo diet plan is a dietary program that mimics the way prehistoric people could eat. It involves the consumption of whole foods that people could scavenge or gather.

Paleo diet plan promoters reject new diet programs that are usually full of processed foods. They think that the time of how hunter-gatherers consumed might cause fewer health problems.

The paleo diet plan is not safe for everyone. Doctors have no idea about its results on children, pregnant women, or older adults. Individuals with persistent problems, such as inflammatory bowel disease, should talk to a doctor before trying a paleo diet plan. This manual explores paleo principles and a 7-day paleo diet meal to follow. Read on to understand how to consume like our ancestors. The paleo diet plan focuses on consuming foods that may have been obtainable as early as the Paleolithic era.

Additionally, the paleo diet plan is called the rock age diet plan, hunter-gatherer diet plan, or caveman diet plan. Before contemporary agriculture developed about 10,000 years ago, people usually ate foods they could hunt or gather, such as fish, liver organs, fruits, vegetables, peanuts, and seeds. The introduction of modern agriculture changed the way people ate. Dairy products, dry beans, and grains became a part of people's food plans.

Proponents of the paleo diet plan believe that the body did not evolve to process dairy, dry beans, and grains. Consuming these foods could increase the threat of specific health problems, such as cardiovascular disease, overweight, and diabetes.

Health advantages of paleo

Individuals state that the paleo eating plan offers numerous health advantages, such as promoting weight reduction, reducing the possibility of diabetes, and decreasing blood pressure. In this area, we review the scientific evidence to find out what studies facilitate these claims:

Excess weight loss

A 2008 research study found that 14 healthy volunteers achieved an average weight reduction of 2.3 pounds by following a paleo diet plan for three weeks.

In 2009, researchers compared the consequences of the paleo diet plan with the diabetes diet plan on 13 people with type 2 diabetes. A little research discovered that consuming the paleo method decreased the individuals' body weight and waist area. The 2014 research on 70 post-menopausal women with weight problems found that executing a paleo diet plan helped individual lose weight after six months.

However, right after 24 months, there was simply no difference in weight reduction between individuals following a paleo diet and those following regular Nordic nutritional suggestions. These findings state that some other healthy diet programs could be just as effective in advertising weight reduction.

The authors of the 2017 review noted that this paleo diet plan helped reduce weight for a while, but they understood that this result was due to calorie restriction or eating fewer calories. Overall, the study shows that the paleo diet plan can help people lose weight initially, but that other diet plans that reduce calorie consumption could be effective. Also, the study is essential before doctors recommend the paleo diet plan for weight reduction. Currently, doctors recommend following exercise and a calorie-controlled diet even more to lose excess weight.

Decrease the risk of diabetes

Does running a paleo diet program reduce the danger of getting diabetes? The results of some preliminary research are usually encouraging. The level of insulin resistance is a dangerous element of diabetes. Improving one's level of insulin sensitivity reduces the likelihood of leading to diabetes and helps those with diabetes decrease signs and symptoms. A 2015 study compared the consequences of the paleo diet plan with those of a diet plan based on the American Diabetes Association's recommendations on people who have type 2 diabetes. While both diet plans improved individuals' metabolic health, the paleo diet plan improved insulin resistance and control of blood sugar levels. A 2009 study of nine sedentary volunteers without obesity found that the paleo diet plan improved insulin awareness.

There is a need for a more recent study on the paleo diet plan and diabetes. However, the evidence so far shows that eating just like a hunter-gatherer can improve insulin sensitivity.

Decrease blood pressure

Increased blood pressure is a factor that leads to the onset of cardiovascular disease. Many believe that the paleo eating plan can help keep blood pressure balanced and increase coronary artery wellness.

A 2010 research on 14 healthy volunteers found that following a paleo eating plan for three weeks improved systolic blood pressure. It additionally reduced excess weight and body mass catalog (BMI). The analysis does not add a group of handles, and yet the results are usually not conclusive. A 2017 research reported results similar to the first ones obtained. Researchers compared the consequences of the paleo diet plan with those of a diet plan that Dutch well-being authorities recommend on 48 individuals with characteristics of metabolic symptoms, a disorder that increases the danger of cardiovascular disease.

The results showed how the paleo diet plan reduced blood pressure and liver lipid levels, both of which can improve body wellness.

Although preliminary studies state that the paleo diet can reduce blood pressure and support heart health, more recent supporting studies will be essential to conclude.

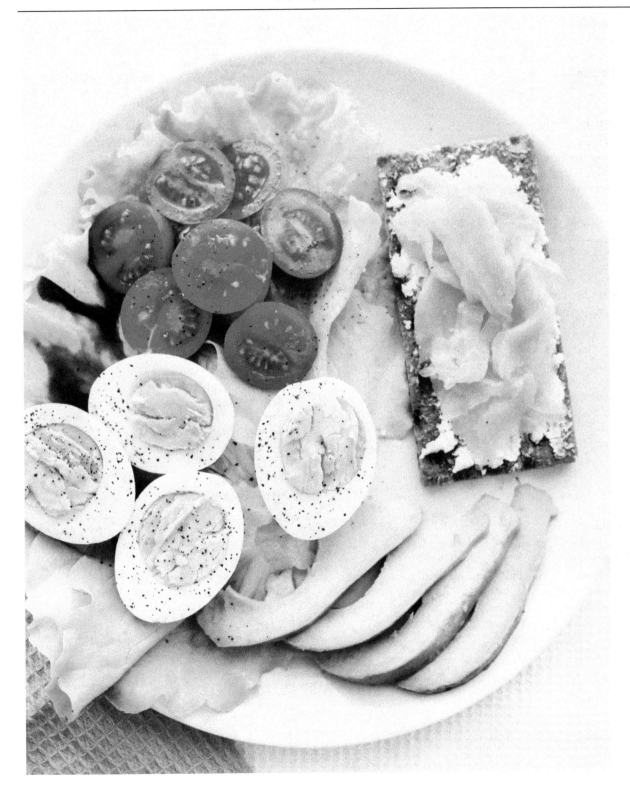

1) Easy Salmon Sheet Pan Dinner

Preparation Time: 30 minutes

Servings: 4

Ingredients:

- ✓ 1 1/2 cups cherry tomatoes
- ✓ 1 large fennel bulb, sliced lengthwise into steaks
- ✓ 1 zucchini, cut into coins

Ingredients:

- ✓ olive oil
- ✓ 2 lemons, halved
- ✓ 1 1/2 pounds salmon filet, whole or cut into filets
- ✓ kosher salt, to taste

Directions:

- ❖ Preheat oven to 450 degrees F.
- ❖ Place the first 5 ingredients on a sheet pan and toss with olive oil to coat and salt to taste.
- ❖ Distribute the vegetables around the pan in a single layer and bake for 10 minutes.
- ❖ Remove the sheet pan from the oven and push some of the vegetables to the side to make space for the salmon fillets.

- ❖ Season the salmon with salt and bake for 12-15 additional minutes (depending on the thickness of your salmon fillets).
- ❖ Turn the broiler on for 2 minutes or until the vegetables are golden.
- ❖ Place salmon and vegetables on a plate and offer a lemon half for squeezing over fish and vegetables.

2) Delicious Turkey Zucchini Burgers with Yogurt-Sumac Sauce

Preparation Time: 20 minutes

Servings: 4

Ingredients:

- ✓ For the burgers:
- ✓ 1 pound ground turkey, light or dark meat
- ✓ 1 large zucchini, coarsely grated
- ✓ 3 scallions, thinly sliced
- ✓ 1 large egg
- ✓ 2 tbsps chopped mint
- ✓ 2 tbsp chopped cilantro
- ✓ 2 garlic cloves, minced
- ✓ 1 tsp ground cumin

Ingredients:

- ✓ 1 teaspoon kosher salt
- ✓ olive oil, for greasing the pan
- ✓ 8 mini hamburger buns
- ✓ For the yogurt sauce:
- ✓ 1 cup greek yogurt
- ✓ 1 teaspoon grated lemon zest
- ✓ 1 tbsp lemon juice
- ✓ 1 garlic clove, minced
- ✓ 1 tbsp olive oil
- ✓ 2 teaspoons sumac
- ✓ 1/2 teaspoon kosher salt

Directions:

- ❖ In a large bowl combine first 9 ingredients.
- ❖ Mix well.
- ❖ With dampened hands form the mixture into burgers about 1 inch thick. You can do small slider size or regular size burgers.

- ❖ In a large saute pan or stove top grill over medium, add 1-2 tbsps olive oil and add the burger patties.
- ❖ Cook burgers 3-4 minutes on each side for small slider burgers or 5-6 minutes on each side for larger burgers.
- ❖ Place all the sauce ingredients in a small bowl and stir to combine.
- ❖ Place the burgers on buns and top with the yogurt-sumac sauce.

3) Special Hearty Breakfast

Preparation Time: 35 minutes

Servings: 2

Ingredients:

- ✓ 3 lb. pork roast, boneless
- ✓ 2 tsp. cumin, ground
- ✓ 1 tsp. red pepper flakes, crushed
- ✓ A pinch of sea salt and black pepper
- ✓ 1 tsp. oregano, dried
- ✓ Juice from 1 orange
- ✓ Orange peel from 1 orange, grated

Directions:

- ❖ Put roast in your instant pot.
- ❖ Add cumin, pepper flakes, salt, pepper, oregano, orange juice, orange peel, garlic, yellow onion, bay leaf and oil and rub roast well.
- ❖ Cover instant pot and cook on high for 20 minutes.

Nutrition: Calories275 | Fat: 4g | Carbs: 5g | Protein: 14g | Fiber: 3g | Sugar: 0g

Ingredients:

- ✓ 6 garlic cloves, minced
- ✓ 1 yellow onion, chopped
- ✓ 1 bay leaf
- ✓ 1 tbsp. avocado oil
- ✓ 2 tsp. cilantro, chopped
- ✓ 1 butter lettuce head, torn
- ✓ 2 radishes, sliced
- ✓ 2 avocados, pitted, peeled and sliced
- ✓ 1 cup Paleo salsa
- ✓ 2 jalapeños, chopped
- ✓ 3 limes, quartered
- ❖ Transfer roast to a cutting board, leave aside to cool down a bit, shred and divide among plates.
- ❖ Also divide lettuce leaves, radishes, avocado slices, jalapeños and lime wedges.
- ❖ Sprinkle cilantro, divide salsa on top and serve for breakfast.

4) **Easy Breakfast Quiche**

Preparation Time: 30 minutes

Servings: 2

Ingredients:

- ✓ 1 cup water
- ✓ 6 eggs, whisked
- ✓ A pinch of black pepper
- ✓ ½ cup coconut milk

Directions:

- ❖ Put the water in your instant pot and add the steamer basket inside.
- ❖ Put bacon, sausage and ham in a bowl, mix and spread on the bottom of a quiche dish.

Ingredients:

- ✓ 4 bacon slices, cooked and crumbled
- ✓ 1 cup sausage, cooked and ground
- ✓ ½ cup ham, chopped
- ✓ 2 green onions, chopped
- ❖ In a bowl, mix eggs with black pepper, coconut milk and green onions and whisk well.
- ❖ Pour this over meat, spread, place inside the pot, cover and cook on high for 30 minutes
- ❖ Slice, divide among plates and serve.

Nutrition: Calories243 | Fat: 3g | Carbs: 6g | Protein: 12g | Fiber: 1g | Sugar: 0g

5) Wonderful Omelette

Preparation Time: 18 minutes   **Servings: 2**

Ingredients:

- ✓ 4 oz. sweet potatoes, cut into medium fries
- ✓ 6 eggs
- ✓ A pinch of sea salt and black pepper
- ✓ 1 tbsp. olive oil
- ✓ ¼ cup scallions, chopped

Directions:

- ❖ Grease a heat proof dish with the oil and spread sweet potato fries on the bottom.
- ❖ In a bowl, mix eggs with salt, pepper, scallions, garlic and bell pepper and whisk well.
- ❖ In another bowl, mix coconut milk with tomato paste and stir.

Ingredients:

- ✓ 1 garlic clove, minced
- ✓ ¼ cup coconut milk
- ✓ 1 tsp. Paleo tomato paste
- ✓ 1 and ½ cups water
- ✓ 1 green bell pepper, chopped
- ❖ Pour this over eggs mix, stir well and spread everything on top of sweet potato fries.
- ❖ Put the water in your instant pot, add the steamer basket inside and place the eggs mix in the basket.
- ❖ Cover, cook on high for 18 minutes, slice, divide among plates and serve hot.

Nutrition: Calories153 | Fat: 7g | Carbs: 5g | Protein: 15g | Fiber: 2g | Sugar: 0g

6) Special Pumpkin and Apple Butter

Preparation Time: 10 minutes   **Servings: 2**

Ingredients:

- ✓ 3 apples, peeled, cored and chopped
- ✓ 30 oz. pumpkin puree
- ✓ 1 tbsp. pumpkin pie spice

Directions:

- ❖ Put pumpkin puree in your instant pot.
- ❖ Add apples, pumpkin pie spice, cider and honey, stir well, cover and cook on high for 10 minutes

Ingredients:

- ✓ 1 cup honey
- ✓ 12 oz. apple cider

- ❖ Divide into jars, seal them and serve for breakfast when ever you want.

Nutrition: Calories100 | Fat: 3g | Carbs: 4g | Protein: 6g | Fiber: 1g | Sugar: 0g

7) Easy Breakfast Spinach Delight

Preparation Time: 30 minutes   **Servings: 2**

Ingredients:

- ✓ 1 lb. mustard leaves
- ✓ 1 lb. spinach, torn
- ✓ 2 tbsp. olive oil
- ✓ A small ginger piece, grated
- ✓ 2 yellow onions, chopped
- ✓ 4 garlic cloves, minced
- ✓ 1 tsp. cumin, ground

Directions:

- ❖ Set your instant pot on sauté mode, add oil and heat it up.
- ❖ Add onion, garlic, ginger, coriander, cumin, garam masala, turmeric, cayenne pepper, black pepper and fenugreek, stir and cook for 5 minutes.

Ingredients:

- ✓ 1 tsp. coriander, ground
- ✓ 1 tsp. garam masala
- ✓ A pinch of cayenne pepper
- ✓ ½ tsp. turmeric
- ✓ A pinch of black pepper
- ✓ A pinch of fenugreek leaves, dried

- ❖ Add spinach and mustard leaves, stir gently, cover and cook on high for 15 minutes.
- ❖ Divide into bowls and serve for breakfast.

Nutrition: Calories200 | Fat: 3g | Carbs: 5g | Protein: 7g | Fiber: 2g | Sugar: 0g

8) Special and Amazing Bacon and Sweet Potato Breakfast

Preparation Time: 10 minutes

Servings: 2

Ingredients:

- ✓ 2 lbs. sweet potatoes, cubed
- ✓ A pinch of salt and black pepper
- ✓ 3 bacon strips

Ingredients:

- ✓ 2 tbsp. water
- ✓ 2 tsp. parsley, dried
- ✓ 1 tsp. garlic powder
- ✓ 4 eggs, fried for serving
- ❖ Divide among plates next to fried eggs and serve.

Directions:

- ❖ In your instant pot, mix sweet potatoes with bacon, salt, pepper, water, parsley and garlic powder, stir, cover and cook on high for 10 minutes.

Nutrition: Calories200 | Fat: 2g | Carbs: 6g | Protein: 8g | Fiber: 2g | Sugar: 0g

9) Easy and Spiced Carrot Cauliflower Soup

Preparation Time: 40 minutes

Servings: 6-8

Ingredients:

- ✓ 1 tbsp olive oil
- ✓ 1 small onion, chopped
- ✓ 5 cups warm water
- ✓ 2 tbsp vegetable bouillon*
- ✓ 1 head cauliflower, chopped (about 4 cups)

Ingredients:

- ✓ 3 cups peeled and chopped carrots (about 8 medium carrots)
- ✓ 1 1/2 tsp curry powder
- ✓ 1 teaspoon ground cinnamon
- ✓ 1 teaspoon garam masala
- ✓ 1 teaspoon kosher salt
- ❖ Bring to a boil, cover, and reduce heat to simmer for 15-20 minutes, or until the vegetables are fork tender.
- ❖ Using an immersion blender or standing blender, puree all of the ingredients until smooth.

Directions:

- ❖ Heat the oil in a large saucepan over medium heat and cook the onions for 3 minutes, or until soft.
- ❖ Dissolve the vegetable bouillon in the water and add to the pot.
- ❖ Add the remaining ingredients to the pot and stir to combine.

10) Special Salmon BLT Salad with Chive Ranch Dressing

Preparation Time: 25 minutes   **Servings: 2-4**

Ingredients:

- ✓ dressing:
- ✓ 1/4 cup plain unsweetened almond milk
- ✓ 1/2 cup paleo mayo homemade or store bought
- ✓ 1 Tbsps lemon juice
- ✓ 1 tsp fresh minced dill or 1/4 tsp dried
- ✓ 1 garlic clove minced
- ✓ 2 Tbsp chopped chives
- ✓ Sea Salt and black pepper to taste
- ✓ Salmon
- ✓ 3/4 tsp sea salt
- ✓ 1/8 tsp black pepper

Ingredients:

- ✓ 1 lb individual salmon fillets skin on or off (3-4 fillets)
- ✓ 3/4 tsp garlic powder
- ✓ 3/4 tsp onion powder
- ✓ 3/4 tsp smoked paprika
- ✓ 1 Tbsp bacon fat avocado oil, or ghee
- ✓ salad:
- ✓ 6 cups mixed greens of choice roughly chopped
- ✓ 1 cup cherry tomatoes halved
- ✓ 6 Slices bacon cooked until crisp and crumbled or chopped
- ✓ 1 medium avocado thinly sliced
- ✓ 1 small red onion thinly sliced
- ❖ Add oil to the skillet. In a skillet, place the salmon skin side down (if you chose skin) and cook about 3 minutes on each side, adjusting for preference and thickness.
- ❖ If grilling, brush grill with oil and place the salmon flesh side down on the hot grill.
- ❖ Cook about 3 minutes, then carefully flip and cook skin side down for another 3-4 minutes, adjusting for thickness and preference.
- ❖ Remove to a plate and assemble the salad.
- ❖ Layer the greens with tomatoes, bacon, sliced avocado and red onion and place salmon on top.
- ❖ Drizzle all over with as much of the dressing as you like and garnish with extra chives if desired. Serve right away. Enjoy!

Directions:

- ❖ dressing:
- ❖ Whisk together the almond milk, mayo, lemon juice and dill until smooth.
- ❖ Stir in the garlic and chives, then season to taste with sea salt and black pepper.
- ❖ salmon:
- ❖ Pat the fillets dry with paper towel. In a small bowl, mix together all the seasonings. You can make the salmon on the stovetop in a skillet or on the grill. If grilling, brush generously all over with the oil before beginning. If pan frying, the oil is for the skillet.
- ❖ Heat the grill or skillet to medium high heat.

11) Easy Garlic Butter Steak Bites

Preparation Time: 20 minutes

Servings: 2-4

Ingredients:

- ✓ ½ tbsp avocado oil
- ✓ 2 pounds of steak, cut into small bite size pieces
- ✓ 2 teaspoons salt
- ✓ ½ teaspoon freshly ground black pepper

Directions:

- ❖ Season the steak bites with salt, pepper, and red pepper flakes and stir until well coated.
- ❖ Heat a large skillet over medium-high heat.
- ❖ Add the avocado oil to the hot skillet and then add the steak in a single layer.
- ❖ Cook the steak bites for 3-4 minutes until brown, stirring occasionally. You may have to do this in batches depending on the size of your skillet.

Ingredients:

- ✓ ½ teaspoon red pepper flakes (optional)
- ✓ 2 tbsps butter or ghee
- ✓ 6 cloves minced garlic
- ✓ ¼ cup chopped parsley
- ✓ green onion, for garnish
- ❖ Once the steak is brown, remove it from the pan.
- ❖ Remove any excess water from the skillet and then add the butter or ghee to the pan.
- ❖ Next add the garlic and saute for 1 minute.
- ❖ Add the steak back to the pan and cook for 1-2 minutes stirring to coat it in the butter sauce.
- ❖ Remove the pan from the heat and stir in the chopped parsley.
- ❖ Garnish with green onion and serve immediately.

12) Special Shrimp Fried Cauliflower Rice

Preparation Time: 25 minutes

Servings: 2-4

Ingredients:

- ✓ 1 lb medium-large raw shrimp peeled and deveined
- ✓ 1 tsp tapioca flour or arrowroot*
- ✓ Sea salt and black pepper
- ✓ 2 Tbsp avocado oil or ghee divided
- ✓ 3 eggs whisked
- ✓ 1 1/2 cups carrots diced
- ✓ 1 bunch scallions white and green parts separated - thinly sliced

Directions:

- ❖ Have all ingredients prepped and ready to go before beginning.
- ❖ In a bowl, toss the shrimp with the tapioca or arrowroot, salt and pepper. Heat a large nonstick skillet over medium high heat.
- ❖ Once hot, add 1 Tbsp avocado oil or ghee.
- ❖ Add shrimp in a single layer and cook 1-2 minutes per side until opaque, careful not to overcook.
- ❖ Remove to a plate and turn the heat to medium.
- ❖ With the skillet over medium heat, add the whisked eggs and cook until just set, breaking them up with your spatula.
- ❖ Set them aside with the shrimp.
- ❖ Add the second tbsp of oil or ghee to the skillet and adjust heat medium high.

Ingredients:

- ✓ 1 inch chunk fresh ginger peeled and minced about 2 tsp
- ✓ 3 cloves garlic minced
- ✓ 12 oz cauliflower rice fresh or frozen. If frozen, thaw first.
- ✓ 1/4 cup coconut aminos (this is a paleo and Whole30 friendly equivalent of soy sauce)
- ✓ 1 tbsp pure sesame oil
- ✓ Sea salt to taste
- ❖ Add the diced carrots and cook, stirring, 3-4 minutes or until fork tender.
- ❖ Then add in the white part of the scallions, ginger, and garlic and stir to combine.
- ❖ Cook another minute until fragrant.
- ❖ Add in the cauliflower rice, coconut aminos and sesame oil and stir to combine.
- ❖ Cook about 2-3 minutes to soften the cauliflower rice.
- ❖ Add in the shrimp and eggs and stir and cook 30-60 seconds to heat through, then remove from heat.
- ❖ Garnish with the green part of the scallions and additional coconut aminos or salt and pepper to taste.
- ❖ Serve right away. Leftovers can be saved in the sealed container in the refrigerator for up to 4 days. Enjoy

13) Special Thai Chicken Satay

Preparation Time: 30 minutes

Servings: 2-4

Ingredients:

- ✓ Thai chicken satay marinade:
- ✓ 1.5-2 lbs chicken thighs, boneless and skinless
- ✓ 1 tsp turmeric powder
- ✓ 1 tsp coriander powder
- ✓ 0.5 tsp white pepper
- ✓ 0.5 tsp cumin powder

Ingredients:

- ✓ 4 tbsp dairy-free coffee creamer, or melted coconut cream
- ✓ 1 tsp fish sauce
- ✓ 2 tbsp coconut aminos, or 1 tbsp low sodium/gluten-free tamari
- ✓ 2 tsp grated ginger
- ✓ 2 tbsp hot sauce, I use Frank's original hot sauce
- ✓ Avocado oil cooking spray, for the air fryer basket
- ❖ Air fry at 370F (188C) for 15 minutes on the first side and 8-10 minutes the second side or until the chicken is cooked through. Please note that cook time varies, depending on the type of air fryer.

Directions:

- ❖ In a large mixing bowl, marinate the chicken thighs with ingredients from turmeric to hot sauce.
- ❖ Gently mix well and cover the bowl.
- ❖ Store in the fridge for at least 30 minutes or up to 1 day before cooking.
- ❖ To air fry, lightly spray the fryer basket with avocado oil.
- ❖ Slightly drip off the marinade and place the chicken thighs into the basket in one layer with some space between each piece.
- ❖ Please do not over crowd the basket. I cook mine in two batches.

- ❖ To pan fry (stovetop), add 1 tbsp avocado oil to a well-heated skillet.
- ❖ Pan fry 6 minutes the first side and 5-6 minutes the second side over medium heat or until the chicken is cooked through.
- ❖ Serve hot or at room temperature. The chicken is very tender and flavorful and you don't need a dipping sauce however if you like to kick the flavor over the top, try my Paleo Thai "Peanut" sauce.
- ❖ Serve it over a big bowl of salad greens or Keto garlic fried rice!

14) Special Morning Berry-Green Smoothie

Preparation Time: 5 minutes

Servings: 4

Ingredients:

- ✓ 3 cups mixed blueberries and strawberries
- ✓ 1 avocado, pitted and sliced
- ✓ 2 cups unsweetened almond milk

Ingredients:

- ✓ 6 tbsp heavy cream
- ✓ 2 tbsp erythritol
- ✓ 1 cup ice cubes
- ✓ ⅓ cup nuts and seeds mix
- ❖ Blend at high speed until smooth and uniform. Pour the smoothie into drinking glasses and serve immediately.

Directions:

- ❖ Combine the avocado slices, blueberries, strawberries, almond milk, heavy cream, erythritol, ice cubes, nuts, and seeds in a smoothie maker.

Nutrition: Calories Calories 360, Fat 33.3g, Net Carbs 6g, Protein 6g

15) Nut Granola and Smoothie Bowl

Preparation Time: 5 minutes

Servings: 4

Ingredients:

- ✓ 6 cups Greek yogurt
- ✓ 4 tbsp almond butter
- ✓ A handful toasted walnuts

Ingredients:

- ✓ 3 tbsp unsweetened cocoa powder
- ✓ 4 tsp swerve brown sugar
- ✓ 2 cups nut granola for topping
- ❖ Share the smoothie into four breakfast bowls, top with a half cup of granola each one, and serve.

Directions:

- ❖ Combine the Greek yogurt, almond butter, walnuts, cocoa powder, and swerve brown sugar in a smoothie maker. Puree at high speed until smooth and well mixed

Nutrition: Calories 361K, Fat 31.2g, Net Carbs 2g, Protein 13g

16) Morning Almond Shake

Preparation Time: 5 minutes

Servings: 2

Ingredients:

- ✓ 1 ½ cups almond milk
- ✓ 2 tbsp almond butter
- ✓ ½ tsp almond extract
- ✓ ½ tsp cinnamon

Ingredients:

- ✓ 2 tbsp flax meal
- ✓ 1 tbsp collagen peptides
- ✓ A pinch of salt
- ✓ 15 drops of stevia
- ✓ A handful of ice cubes
- ❖ Then taste and adjust flavor as needed, adding more stevia for sweetness or almond butter to the creaminess. Pour in a smoothie glass, add the ice cubes and sprinkle with cinnamon.

Directions:

- ❖ Add almond milk, almond butter, flax meal, almond extract, collagen peptides, a pinch of salt, and stevia to a blender bowl. Blitz until uniform and smooth, about 30 seconds.

Nutrition: Calories Calories 326, Fat: 27g, Net Carbs: 6g, Protein: 19g

17) Delicious Chocolate Protein Coconut Shake

Preparation Time: 5 minutes

Servings: 4

Ingredients:

- ✓ 3 cups flax milk, chilled
- ✓ 3 tsp unsweetened cocoa powder
- ✓ 1 medium avocado, peeled, sliced
- ✓ 1 cup coconut milk, chilled

Ingredients:

- ✓ 3 mint leaves + extra to garnish
- ✓ 3 tbsp erythritol
- ✓ 1 tbsp low carb protein powder
- ✓ Whipping cream for topping
- ❖ Pour the drink into serving glasses, lightly add some whipping cream on top, and garnish with 1 or 2 mint leaves. Serve immediately.

Directions:

- ❖ Combine the flax milk, cocoa powder, avocado, coconut milk, 3 mint leaves, erythritol, and protein powder into the smoothie maker, and blend for 1 minute to smooth.

Nutrition: Calories Calories 265, Fat: 15.5g, Net Carbs: 4g, Protein: 12g

18) Easy Five Greens Smoothie

Preparation Time: 5 minutes

Servings: 4

Ingredients:

- ✓ 6 kale leaves, chopped
- ✓ 3 stalks celery, chopped
- ✓ 1 ripe avocado, skinned and sliced

Directions:

- ❖ In a blender, add the kale, celery, avocado, and ice cubes, and blend for 45 seconds. Add the spinach and cucumber, and process for another 45 seconds until smooth

Ingredients:

- ✓ 2 cups spinach, chopped
- ✓ 1 cucumber, peeled and chopped
- ✓ Chia seeds to garnish
- ❖ Pour the smoothie into glasses, garnish with chia seeds, and serve the drink immediately.

Nutrition: Calories Calories 124, Fat 7.8g, Net Carbs 2.9g, Protein 3.2g

19) Special Dark Chocolate Smoothie

Preparation Time: 10 minutes

Servings: 2

Ingredients:

- ✓ ½ cup pecans
- ✓ ¾ cup coconut milk
- ✓ ¼ cup water
- ✓ 4 oz watercress

Directions:

- ❖ In a blender, add all ingredients and process until creamy and uniform.

Ingredients:

- ✓ 1 tsp low carb protein powder
- ✓ 1 tbsp chia seeds
- ✓ 1 tbsp unsweetened cocoa powder
- ✓ 4 fresh dates, pitted
- ❖ Chill and serve in glasses

Nutrition: Calories Calories 335; Fat: 31.7g Net Carbs: 12.7g, Protein: 7g

20) Special Bacon and Egg Quesadillas

Preparation Time: 30 minutes

Servings: 4

Ingredients:

- ✓ 8 low carb tortilla shells
- ✓ 6 eggs
- ✓ 1 cup water
- ✓ 3 tbsp butter

Directions:

- ❖ Bring the eggs to a boil in water over medium heat for 10 minutes. Transfer the eggs to an ice water bath, peel the shells, and chop them. Fry the bacon in a skillet over medium heat for 4 minutes until crispy. Remove and chop. Sauté the onion in the remaining grease 2 minutes; set aside.
- ❖ Melt 1 tbsp of butter in another skillet over medium heat. Lay one tortilla in a skillet and sprinkle with some Swiss cheese

Ingredients:

- ✓ 1 ½ cups grated cheddar cheese
- ✓ 1 ½ cups grated Swiss cheese
- ✓ 5 bacon slices
- ✓ 1 medium onion, thinly sliced
- ✓ 1 tbsp parsley, chopped
- ❖ Add some chopped eggs and bacon over the cheese, top with onion, and sprinkle with some cheddar cheese. Cover with another tortilla shell. Cook for 45 seconds
- ❖ Carefully flip the quesadilla, and cook the other side too for 45 seconds. Remove to a plate and repeat the cooking process using the remaining tortilla shells. Garnish with parsley and serve warm.

Nutrition: Calories Calories 449, Fat 48.7g, Net Carbs 6.8g, Protein 29.1g

21) Delicious Almond Waffles with Cinnamon Cream

Preparation Time: 25 minutes

Servings: 6

Ingredients:

✓ Cinnamon cream
✓ 8 oz cream cheese, softened
✓ 1 tsp cinnamon powder
✓ 3 tbsp swerve brown sugar
✓ 2 tbsp cinnamon

Ingredients:

✓ Waffles
✓ 5 tbsp butter, melted
✓ 1 ½ cups unsweetened almond milk
✓ 7 large eggs
✓ ¼ tsp liquid stevia
✓ ½ tsp baking powder
✓ 1 ½ cups almond flour
❖ Let the batter sit for 5 minutes to thicken. Spritz a waffle iron with a cooking spray.
❖ Ladle a ¼ cup of the batter into the waffle iron and cook according to the manufacturer's instructions until golden, about 10 minutes in total. Repeat with the remaining batter. Slice the waffles into quarters. Apply the cinnamon spread in between each of two waffles and snap. Serve.

Directions:

❖ Combine cream cheese, cinnamon, and swerve with a mixer until smooth. Cover and chill until ready to use.
❖ To make the waffles, whisk the butter, milk, and eggs in a medium bowl. Add the stevia and baking powder and mix. Stir in the almond flour and combine until no lumps exist

Nutrition: Calories Calories 307, Fat 24g, Net Carbs 8g, Protein 12g

22) Special Cajun Shrimp and Sausage Skillets

Preparation Time: 20 minutes

Servings: 2-4

Ingredients:

✓ 2 tablespoons avocado oil or ghee
✓ 12 oz andouille sausage, sliced
✓ 1 tbsp finely minced garlic
✓ 1 small red bell pepper, sliced
✓ 1 small green bell pepper, sliced
✓ salt and pepper to taste

Directions:

❖ Heat a large skillet over medium-high heat.
❖ Once the skillet is hot, add in the avocado oil or ghee.
❖ Add the minced garlic and cook for minute until fragrant.
❖ Add the sliced andouille sausage and cook for three to four minutes to brown on both sides.
❖ When the sausage has browned, add the sliced bell peppers and onions to the skillet.

Ingredients:

✓ 1 small orange bell pepper, sliced
✓ 1/2 yellow onion, sliced
✓ 1/4 cup sliced green onion
✓ 1 pound shrimp, peeled and deveined
✓ 1/2 tablespoon cajun seasoning (plus more to taste)
✓ juice of one lemon
❖ Season with salt, pepper, and the cajun seasoning. Cook the veggies for three to four minutes.
❖ Next, add the shrimp to the skillet and toss to combine.
❖ Cook for two to three minutes until the shrimp is translucent and cooked through.
❖ Remove the skillet from the heat and add the lemon juice, sliced green onion, and more seasoning to taste.
❖ Serve immediately.

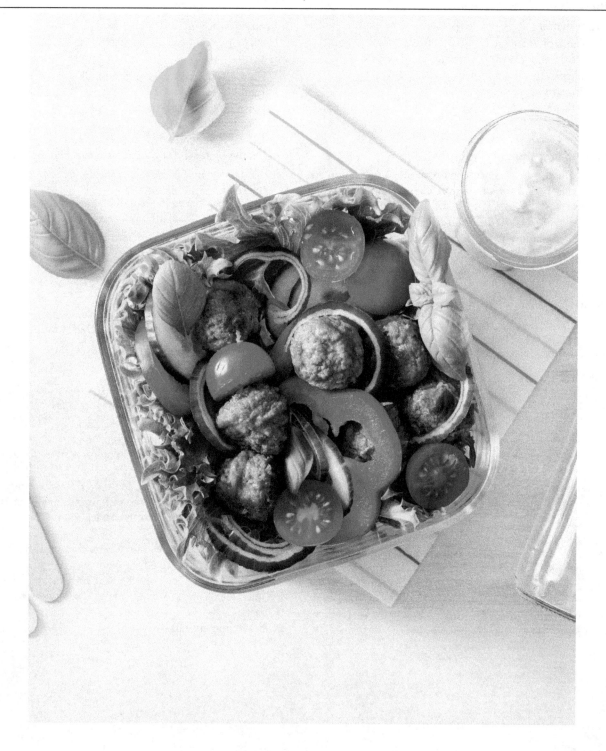

23) Special and Sweet Chili Grilled Chicken

Preparation Time: 30 minutes

Servings: 6

Ingredients:

- ✓ 2 lb chicken breasts
- ✓ 4 cloves garlic, minced
- ✓ 2 tbsp fresh oregano, chopped
- ✓ ½ cup lemon juice

Ingredients:

- ✓ 2/3 cup olive oil
- ✓ 1 tbsp erythritol
- ✓ Salt and black pepper to taste
- ✓ 3 small chilies, minced
- ❖ Remove the wrap and brush the spice mixture on the chicken on all sides. Place on the grill and cook for 15 minutes, flip, and continue cooking for 10 more minutes. Remove to a plate and serve with salad.

Directions:

- ❖ Preheat grill to high heat. In a bowl, mix the garlic, oregano, lemon juice, olive oil, chilies, and erythritol. Cover the chicken with plastic wraps and use the rolling pin to pound to ½-inch thickness.

Nutrition: Calories 265, Fat 9g, Net Carbs 3g, Protein 26g

24) Easy Chicken and Squash Traybake

Preparation Time: 50 minutes

Servings: 4

Ingredients:

- ✓ 1 ½ lb chicken thighs
- ✓ 1 lb butternut squash, cubed
- ✓ ½ cup black olives, pitted

Ingredients:

- ✓ ¼ cup olive oil
- ✓ 5 garlic cloves, sliced
- ✓ ¼ tbsp dried oregano
- ❖ Drizzle with olive oil. Sprinkle with black pepper, salt, and oregano. Bake in the oven for 45 minutes until golden brown. Serve warm.

Directions:

- ❖ Preheat oven to 400°F. Place the chicken in a greased baking dish with the skin down. Place the garlic, olives, and butternut squash around the chicken.

Nutrition: Calories: 411, Fat: 15g, Net Carbs: 5.5g, Protein: 31g

25) Bell Pepper and Beef Sausage Omelette

Preparation Time: approx. 60 minutes

Servings: 4

Ingredients:

- ✓ 12 whole eggs
- ✓ 1 cup sour cream
- ✓ 1 tbsp butter

Ingredients:

- ✓ 2 red bell peppers, chopped
- ✓ 12 oz ground beef sausage
- ✓ ¼ cup shredded cheddar
- ❖ Flatten the beef on the bottom of skillet, scatter bell peppers on top, pour the egg mixture all over, and scatter the top with cheddar cheese. Put the skillet in the oven and bake for 30 minutes or until the eggs set and the cheddar cheese melts. Remove, slice the frittata, and serve warm with a salad.

Directions:

- ❖ Preheat the oven to 350 F. Crack the eggs into a blender; add the sour cream, salt, and pepper. Process over low speed to mix the ingredients; set aside. Melt butter in a large skillet over medium heat. Add bell peppers and sauté until soft, 6 minutes; set aside. Add the beef sausage and cook until brown, continuously stirring and breaking the lumps into small bits, 10 minutes.

Nutrition: Calories 617; Net Carbs 5g; Fat 50g; Protein 33g

26) Italian Chili Zucchini Beef Lasagna

Preparation Time: approx. 55 minutes

Servings: 4

Ingredients:

- ✓ ½ cup Pecorino Romano cheese
- ✓ 4 yellow zucchini, sliced
- ✓ Salt and black pepper to taste
- ✓ 1 tbsp lard
- ✓ ½ lb ground beef
- ✓ 1 tsp garlic powder
- ✓ 1 tsp onion powder
- ✓ 2 tbsp coconut flour

Ingredients:

- ✓ 1 ½ cups grated mozzarella
- ✓ 2 cups crumbled goat cheese
- ✓ 1 large egg
- ✓ 2 cups marinara sauce
- ✓ 1 tbsp Italian herb seasoning
- ✓ ¼ tsp red chili flakes
- ✓ ¼ cup fresh basil leaves

Directions:

- ❖ Preheat oven to 375 F. Melt the lard in a skillet and cook beef for 10 minutes; set aside. In a bowl, combine garlic powder, onion powder, coconut flour, salt, pepper, mozzarella cheese, half of Pecorino cheese, goat cheese, and egg. Mix Italian herb seasoning and chili flakes with marinara sauce. Make a single layer of the zucchini in a greased baking dish, spread ¼ of the egg mixture on top, and ¼ of the marinara sauce.

- ❖ Repeat the process and top with the remaining Pecorino cheese. Bake in the oven for 20 minutes. Garnish with basil, slice, and serve.

Nutrition: Calories 608; Net Carbs 5.5g; Fat 37g; Protein 52g

27) Easy Tarragon Beef Meatloaf

Preparation Time: approx. 70 minutes

Servings: 4

Ingredients:

- ✓ 2 lb ground beef
- ✓ 3 tbsp flaxseed meal
- ✓ 2 large eggs
- ✓ 2 tbsp olive oil
- ✓ 1 lemon, zested

Ingredients:

- ✓ ¼ cup chopped tarragon
- ✓ ¼ cup chopped oregano
- ✓ 4 garlic cloves, minced

Directions:

- ❖ Preheat the oven to 400 F. Grease a loaf pan with cooking spray. In a bowl, combine beef, salt, pepper, and flaxseed meal; set aside. In another bowl, whisk the eggs with olive oil, lemon zest, tarragon, oregano, and garlic. Pour the mixture onto the beef mix and evenly combine.

- ❖ Spoon the meat mixture into the pan and press to fit in. Bake in oven for 1 hour. Remove the pan, tilt to drain the meat's liquid, and let cool for 5 minutes. Slice, garnish with some lemon slices, and serve with curried cauli rice.

Nutrition: Calories 631; Net Carbs 2.8g; Fat 38g; Protein 64g

28) Italian Broccoli Beef Bake with Pancetta

Preparation Time: approx. 55 minutes

Servings: 4

Ingredients:

- ✓ 1 large broccoli head, cut into florets
- ✓ 6 slices pancetta, chopped
- ✓ 2 tbsp olive oil
- ✓ 1 lb ground beef
- ✓ 2 tbsp butter

Ingredients:

- ✓ 1 cup coconut cream
- ✓ 2 oz cream cheese, softened
- ✓ 1 ¼ cups grated cheddar
- ✓ ¼ cup chopped scallions

Directions:

- ❖ Preheat the oven to 300 F. Fill a pot with water and bring to a boil. Pour in broccoli and blanch for 2 minutes. Drain and set aside. Place pancetta in the pot and fry for 5 minutes. Remove to a plate. Heat oil in the pot and cook the beef until brown for 5-6 minutes. Add in coconut cream, cream cheese, two-thirds of cheddar cheese, salt, and pepper and stir for 7 minutes.

- ❖ Arrange the broccoli florets in a baking dish, pour the beef mixture over, and scatter the top with pancetta and scallions. Bake in the oven until the cheese is bubbly and golden, 20 minutes. Top with the remaining cheddar and bake for 10 more minutes. Serve.

Nutrition: Calories 854; Net Carbs 7.3g; Fat 69g; Protein 51g

29) Slow-Cooking BBQ Beef Sliders

Preparation Time: approx. 12 hours 25 minutes

Servings: 4

Ingredients:

- ✓ 4 zero carb hamburger buns, halved
- ✓ 3 lb chuck roast, boneless
- ✓ 1 tsp onion powder
- ✓ 2 tsp garlic powder
- ✓ 1 tbsp smoked paprika
- ✓ 2 tbsp tomato paste

Ingredients:

- ✓ ¼ cup white vinegar
- ✓ 2 tbsp tamari sauce
- ✓ ½ cup bone broth
- ✓ ¼ cup melted butter
- ✓ Salt and black pepper to taste
- ✓ ¼ cup baby spinach
- ✓ 4 slices cheddar cheese

Directions:

- ❖ Cut the beef into two pieces. In a small bowl, combine salt, pepper, onion and garlic powders, and paprika. Rub the mixture onto beef and place it in a slow cooker. In another bowl, mix tomato paste, vinegar, tamari sauce, broth, and melted butter.

- ❖ Pour over the beef and cook for 4 hours on High. When the beef cooks, shred it using two forks. Divide the spinach between buns, spoon the meat on top, and add a cheddar cheese slice. Serve immediately.

Nutrition: Calories 648; Net Carbs 16g; Fat 27g; Protein 72g

30) Special .Roasted Beef Stacks with Cabbage

Preparation Time: approx. 55 minutes

Servings: 4

Ingredients:
- ✓ 1 head canon cabbage, shredded
- ✓ 1 lb chuck steak, sliced thinly across the grain
- ✓ 3 tbsp coconut flour

Ingredients:
- ✓ ¼ cup olive oil
- ✓ 1 tsp Italian mixed herb blend
- ✓ ½ cup bone broth
- ❖ Sprinkle the Italian herb blend and drizzle again with the remaining olive oil. Roast for 30 minutes. Remove the pan and carefully pour in the broth. Return to the oven and roast further for 10 minutes, until beef cooks through.

Directions:
- ❖ Preheat the oven to 400 F. In a zipper bag, add coconut flour, salt, and pepper. Mix and add the beef slices. Seal the bag and shake to coat. Make little mounds of cabbage. in a greased baking dish. Sprinkle with salt and pepper, and drizzle with some olive oil. Remove the beef strips from the coconut flour mixture, shake off the excess flour, and place 2-3 beef strips on each cabbage mound.

Nutrition: Calories 222; Net Carbs 1.5g; Fat 14g; Protein 18g

31) Easy Savory Portobello Beef Burgers

Preparation Time: approx. 30 minutes

Servings: 4

Ingredients:
- ✓ 4 large Portobello caps, destemmed and rinsed
- ✓ 1 lb ground beef
- ✓ Salt and black pepper to taste
- ✓ 1 tbsp Worcestershire sauce

Ingredients:
- ✓ 1 tbsp coconut oil
- ✓ 4 slices Monterey Jack
- ✓ 4 lettuce leaves
- ✓ 4 large tomato slices
- ✓ ¼ cup mayonnaise
- ❖ Remove to serving plates. Cook the beef patties in the skillet until brown, 10 minutes in total. Place the cheese slices on the beef, allow melting for 1 minute and lift each beef patty onto each mushroom cap. Cover with the lettuce, tomato slices, and mayo and serve.

Directions:
- ❖ In a bowl, combine beef, salt, pepper, and Worcestershire sauce. Using your hands, mold the meat into 4 patties, and set aside. Heat the coconut oil in a skillet over medium heat. Place in the Portobello caps and cook until softened, 4 minutes.

Nutrition: Calories 332; Net Carbs 0.7g; Fat 22g; Protein 29g

32) Rich Spicy Enchilada Beef Stuffed Peppers

Preparation Time: approx. 70 minutes

Servings: 6

Ingredients:

- ✓ 6 bell peppers, deseeded
- ✓ 1 ½ tbsp olive oil
- ✓ 3 tbsp butter, softened
- ✓ ½ white onion, chopped
- ✓ 3 cloves garlic, minced

Ingredients:

- ✓ 2 ½ lb ground beef
- ✓ 3 tsp enchilada seasoning
- ✓ 1 cup cauliflower rice
- ✓ ¼ cup grated cheddar cheese
- ✓ Sour cream for serving
- ❖ Spoon the mixture into the peppers, top with the cheddar cheese, and put the stuffed peppers in a greased baking dish. Bake for 40 minutes. Drop generous dollops of sour cream on the peppers and serve.

Directions:

- ❖ Preheat oven to 400 F. Melt butter in a skillet over medium heat and sauté onion and garlic for 3 minutes. Stir in beef, enchilada seasoning, salt, and pepper. Cook for 10 minutes. Mix in the cauli rice until well incorporated.

Nutrition: Calories 409; Net Carbs 4g; Fat 21g; Protein 45g

33) Simple Spicy Beef Lettuce Wraps

Preparation Time: approx. 20 minutes

Servings: 4

Ingredients:

- ✓ 1 lb chuck steak, sliced thinly against the grain
- ✓ 3 tbsp ghee, divided
- ✓ 1 large white onion, chopped
- ✓ 2 garlic cloves, minced
- ✓ 1 jalapeño pepper, chopped

Ingredients:

- ✓ 2 tsp red curry powder
- ✓ 1 cup cauliflower rice
- ✓ 8 small lettuce leaves
- ✓ ¼ cup sour cream for topping

- ❖ Lay out the lettuce leaves on a lean flat surface and spoon the beef mixture onto the middle part of them, 3 tbsp per leaf. Top with sour cream, wrap the leaves, and serve.

Directions:

- ❖ Melt 2 tbsp of ghee in a large deep skillet; season the beef and cook until brown and cooked within, 10 minutes; set aside. Sauté the onion for 3 minutes. Pour in garlic, salt, pepper, and jalapeño and cook for 1 minute.
- ❖ Add the remaining ghee, curry powder, and beef. Cook for 5 minutes and stir in the cauliflower rice. Sauté until adequately mixed and the cauliflower is slightly softened, 2 to 3 minutes. Adjust the taste with salt and black pepper.

Nutrition: Calories 298; Net Carbs 3.3g; Fat 18g; Protein 27g

34) Saturday Beef Sausage Pizza

Preparation Time: approx. 45 minutes

Servings: 4

Ingredients:

- ✓ 2 tbsp cream cheese, softened
- ✓ 6 oz shredded cheese
- ✓ ¾ cup almond flour
- ✓ 1 egg
- ✓ 1 tsp plain vinegar
- ✓ 2 tbsp butter

Ingredients:

- ✓ 8 oz ground beef sausage
- ✓ ¼ cup tomato sauce
- ✓ ½ tsp dried basil
- ✓ 4 ½ oz shredded mozzarella

Directions:

- ❖ Preheat oven to 400 F. Line a pizza pan with parchment paper. Melt cream and mozzarella cheeses in a skillet while stirring until evenly combined. Turn the heat off and mix in almond flour, egg, and vinegar. Let cool slightly.
- ❖ Flatten the mixture onto the pizza pan. Cover with another parchment paper and using a rolling pin, smoothen the dough into a circle. Take off the parchment paper on top, prick the dough all over with a fork and bake for 10 to 15 minutes until golden brown.

- ❖ While the crust bakes, melt butter in a skillet over and fry sausage until brown, 8 minutes. Turn the heat off. Spread the tomato sauce on the crust, top with basil, meat, and mozzarella cheese, and return to the oven. Bake for 12 minutes. Remove the pizza, slice, and serve warm.

Nutrition: Calories 361; Net Carbs 0.8g; Fat 21g; Protein 37g

35) Special Peanut Zucchini and Beef Pad Thai

Preparation Time: approx. 35 minutes

Servings: 4

Ingredients:

- ✓ 2 ½ lb chuck steak, sliced thinly against the grain
- ✓ 1 tsp crushed red pepper flakes
- ✓ 1 tsp freshly pureed garlic
- ✓ ¼ tsp freshly ground ginger
- ✓ Salt and black pepper to taste
- ✓ 2 tbsp peanut oil
- ✓ 3 large eggs, lightly beaten
- ✓ 1/3 cup beef broth

Ingredients:

- ✓ 3 ¼ tbsp peanut butter
- ✓ 2 tbsp tamari sauce
- ✓ 1 tbsp white vinegar
- ✓ ½ cup chopped green onions
- ✓ 2 garlic cloves, minced
- ✓ 4 zucchinis, spiralized
- ✓ ½ cup bean sprouts
- ✓ ½ cup crushed peanuts
- ❖ . Mix until adequately combined and simmer for 3 minutes. Stir in beef, zucchini, bean sprouts, and eggs. Cook for 1 minute. Garnish with peanuts.

Directions:

- ❖ In a bowl, combine garlic puree, ginger, salt, and pepper. Add in beef and toss to coat. Heat peanut oil in a deep skillet and cook the beef for 12 minutes; transfer to a plate. Pour the eggs to the skillet and scramble for 1 minute; set aside. Reduce the heat and combine broth, peanut butter, tamari sauce, vinegar, green onions, minced garlic, and red pepper flakes.

Nutrition: Calories 425; Net Carbs 3.3g; Fat 40g; Protein 70g

36) Hot Lemon and Spinach Cheeseburgers

Preparation Time: approx. 15 minutes

Servings: 4

Ingredients:

- ✓ 1 large tomato, sliced into 4 pieces and deseeded
- ✓ 1 lb ground beef
- ✓ ½ cup chopped cilantro
- ✓ 1 lemon, zested and juiced
- ✓ Salt and black pepper to taste
- ✓ 1 tsp garlic powder

Directions:

- ❖ Preheat the grill on high heat. In a bowl, add beef, cilantro, lemon zest, juice, salt, pepper, garlic powder, and chili puree. Mix the ingredients until evenly combined. Make 4 patties from the mixture. Grill for 3 minutes on each side. Transfer to a serving plate. Lay 2 spinach leaves side to side in 4 portions on a clean flat surface.

Ingredients:

- ✓ 2 tbsp hot chili puree
- ✓ 16 large spinach leaves
- ✓ 4 tbsp mayonnaise
- ✓ 1 medium red onion, sliced
- ✓ ¼ cup grated Parmesan
- ✓ 1 avocado, halved, sliced
- ❖ Place a beef patty on each and spread 1 tbsp of mayo on top. Add a slice of tomato and onion, sprinkle with some Parmesan cheese, and place avocado on top. Cover with 2 pieces of spinach leaves each. Serve the burgers with cream cheese sauce.

Nutrition: Calories 310; Net Carbs 6.5g; Fat 16g; Protein 29g

37) Easy Herby Beef Meatballs

Preparation Time: approx. 30 minutes

Servings: 4

Ingredients:

- ✓ 1 lb ground beef
- ✓ 1 red onion, finely chopped
- ✓ 2 red bell peppers, chopped
- ✓ 2 garlic cloves, minced
- ✓ 2 tbsp melted butter

Directions:

- ❖ Preheat the oven to 400 F. In a bowl, mix beef, onion, bell peppers, garlic, butter, basil, tamari sauce, salt, pepper, and rosemary. Form 1-inch meatballs from the mixture and place on a greased baking sheet.

Ingredients:

- ✓ 1 tsp dried basil
- ✓ 2 tbsp tamari sauce
- ✓ Salt and black pepper to taste
- ✓ 1 tbsp dried rosemary
- ✓ 1 tbsp olive oil

- ❖ Drizzle olive oil over the beef and bake in the oven for 20 minutes or until the meatballs brown on the outside. Serve garnished with scallions and topped with ranch dressing.

Nutrition: Calories 618; Net Carbs 2.5g; Fat 33g; Protein 74g

38) Paleo and .Keto Burgers

Preparation Time: approx. 15 minutes

Servings: 4

Ingredients:

- ✓ 1 pound ground beef
- ✓ ½ tsp onion powder
- ✓ ½ tsp garlic powder
- ✓ 2 tbsp ghee
- ✓ 1 tsp Dijon mustard

Ingredients:

- ✓ 4 zero carb burger buns
- ✓ ¼ cup mayonnaise
- ✓ 1 tsp Sriracha sauce
- ✓ 4 tbsp coleslaw
- ✓ Salt and black pepper to taste
- ❖ Melt ghee in a skillet and cook the burgers for 3 minutes per side. Serve on buns topped with mayonnaise, sriracha sauce, and coleslaw.

Directions:

- ❖ Mix together beef, onion powder, garlic powder, and mustard in a bowl. Create 4 burgers.

Nutrition: Calories 664; Net Carbs 7.9g; Fat 55g; Protein 39g

39) Special Beef Taco pizza

Preparation Time: approx. 45 minutes

Servings: 4

Ingredients:

- ✓ 2 cups shredded mozzarella
- ✓ 2 tbsp cream cheese, softened
- ✓ 1 egg
- ✓ ¾ cup almond flour
- ✓ 1 lb ground beef
- ✓ 2 tsp taco seasoning
- ✓ ½ cup cheese sauce

Ingredients:

- ✓ 1 cup grated cheddar cheese
- ✓ 1 cup chopped lettuce
- ✓ 1 tomato, diced
- ✓ ¼ cup sliced black olives
- ✓ 1 cup sour cream for topping

Directions:

- ❖ Preheat oven to 390 F. Line a pizza pan with parchment paper. Microwave the mozzarella and cream cheeses for 1 minute. Remove and mix in egg and almond flour. Spread the mixture on the pan and bake for 15 minutes. Put the beef in a pot and cook for 5 minutes. Stir in taco seasoning.

- ❖ Spread the cheese sauce on the crust and top with the meat. Add cheddar cheese, lettuce, tomato, and black olives. Bake until the cheese melts, 5 minutes. Remove the pizza, drizzle sour cream on top, and serve.

Nutrition: Calories 590; Net Carbs 7.9g; Fat 29g; Protein 64g

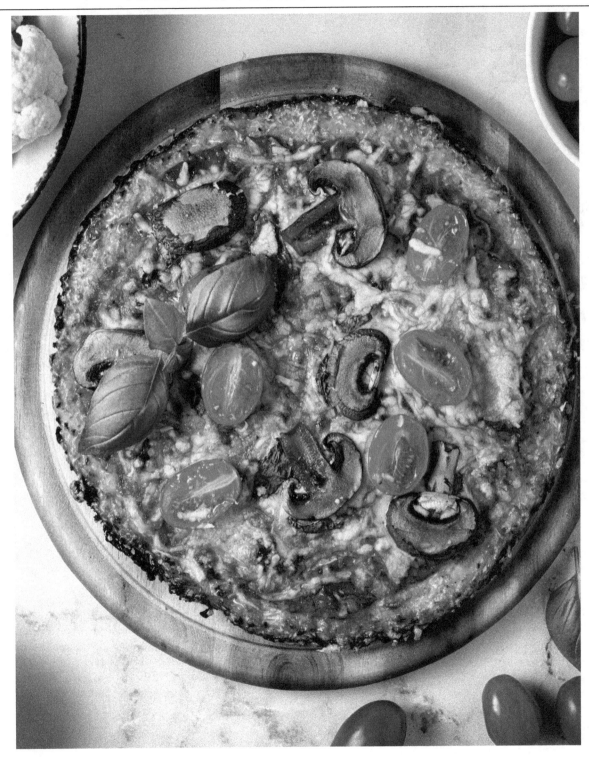

40) Tofu Nuggets with cilantro sauce

Preparation Time: 25 minutes

Servings: 4

Ingredients:

- ✓ 1 lime, ½ squeezed and ½ cut into wedges
- ✓ 1 ½ cups olive oil
- ✓ 28 ounces tofu, pressed and diced
- ✓ 1 egg, lightly beaten
- ✓ 1 cup golden flax seed meal

Directions:

- ❖ Heat the olive oil in a deep skillet. Coat the tofu cubes in the egg and then in the flaxseed meal. Fry until golden brown.

Ingredients:

- ✓ 1 ripe avocado, chopped
- ✓ ½ tbsp chopped cilantro
- ✓ Salt and black pepper to taste
- ✓ ½ tbsp olive oil

- ❖ Transfer to a plate. Place the avocado, cilantro, salt, pepper and lime juice in a blender; blend until smooth. Pour into a bowl, add the tofu nuggets and lime wedges to serve.

Nutrition: Calories 665; Net carbs 6.2g, fat 54g, protein 32g

41) Spicy Brussels sprouts with carrots

Preparation Time: 15 minutes

Servings: 4

Ingredients:

- ✓ 1 pound Brussels sprouts
- ✓ ¼ cup olive oil
- ✓ 4 green onions, chopped

Directions:

- ❖ Sauté green onions in hot olive oil for 2 minutes. Sprinkle with salt and pepper and transfer to a plate. Cut the Brussels sprouts and split them in half.

Ingredients:

- ✓ 2 carrots, grated
- ✓ Salt and black pepper to taste
- ✓ Hot chili sauce
- ❖ Leave the small ones as whole. Pour the Brussels sprouts and carrots into the same saucepan and sauté until softened but al dente. Season to taste and toss with the onions. Cook for 3 minutes. Add chili sauce and serve.

Nutrition: Calories 198; Net carbohydrates 6.5g; Fat 14g; Protein 4.9g

42) Zucchini-Cranberry Cake Squares

Preparation Time: 45 minutes

Servings: 6

Ingredients:

- ✓ 1 ¼ cups chopped zucchini
- ✓ 2 tbsp olive oil
- ✓ ½ cup dried cranberries
- ✓ 1 lemon, peeled
- ✓ 3 eggs

Directions:

- ❖ Preheat oven to 350 F. Line a square cake pan with baking paper. Combine the zucchini, olive oil, cranberries, lemon zest and eggs in a bowl until evenly combined.

Ingredients:

- ✓ 1 ½ cups almond flour
- ✓ ½ tsp baking powder
- ✓ 1 tsp cinnamon powder
- ✓ A pinch of salt

- ❖ Add the almond flour, baking powder, cinnamon powder and salt into the mixture. Pour the mixture into the cake pan and bake for 30 minutes. Remove from the oven, let cool in the cake pan for 10 minutes and transfer the cake to a wire rack to cool completely. Cut into squares and serve.

Nutrition: Calories 121; Net Carbs 2.5g, Fat 10g, Protein 4g

43) Fried rice egg with grilled cheese

Preparation Time: 10 minutes

Servings: 4

Ingredients:
- ✓ 2 cups cauliflower rice, steamed
- ✓ ½ pound halloumi, cut into ¼- to ½-inch slabs
- ✓ 1 tbsp ghee
- ✓ 4 eggs, beaten

Directions:
- ❖ Melt the ghee in a skillet and pour in the eggs. Rotate the pan to scatter the eggs and cook for 1 minute. Move the scrambled eggs to the side of the skillet, add the bell bell pepper and green beans and saute for 3 minutes. Pour in the cauli rice and cook for 2 minutes.

Ingredients:
- ✓ 1 green bell pepper, chopped
- ✓ ¼ cup green beans, chopped
- ✓ 1 tsp soy sauce
- ✓ 2 tbsp chopped parsley
- ❖ Add the soy sauce; combine evenly and cook for 2 minutes. Distribute to plates, garnish with parsley and set aside. Preheat a grill pan and grill halloumi cheese on both sides until cheese turns slightly brown. Place on the side of the rice and serve hot.

Nutrition: Calories 275; Net carbs 4.5g, fat 19g, protein 15g

44) Fake Mushroom Risotto

Preparation Time: 15 minutes

Servings: 4

Ingredients:
- ✓ 2 shallots, diced
- ✓ 3 tbsp olive oil
- ✓ ¼ cup vegetable stock
- ✓ ⅓ cup Parmesan cheese

Directions:
- ❖ Heat 2 tbsp oil in a saucepan, add mushrooms and cook over medium heat for 3 minutes.

Ingredients:
- ✓ 4 tbsp butter
- ✓ 3 tbsp chopped chives
- ✓ 2 pounds mushrooms, sliced
- ✓ 4 1/2 cups rinsed cauliflower
- ❖ Remove and set aside. Heat the remaining oil and cook the shallots for 2 minutes. Add the cauliflower and broth and cook until the liquid is absorbed. Stir in the rest of the ingredients.

Nutrition: Calories 264; Net carbs 8.4g; Fat 18g; Protein 11g

45) Eggplant pizza with cheese

Preparation Time: 40 minutes

Servings: 2

Ingredients:
- ✓ 6 ounces grated mozzarella cheese
- ✓ 2 tbsp cream cheese
- ✓ 2 tbsp Parmesan cheese
- ✓ 1 tsp oregano
- ✓ ½ cup almond flour
- ✓ 2 tbsp psyllium husk

Directions:
- ❖ Preheat oven to 400 F. Melt the mozzarella cheese in the microwave. Combine cream cheese, Parmesan cheese, oregano, almond flour and psyllium husk in a bowl. Add the melted mozzarella cheese and stir to combine.

Ingredients:
- ✓ 4 ounces grated cheddar cheese
- ✓ ¼ cup marinara sauce
- ✓ Eggplant, sliced
- ✓ 1 tomato, sliced
- ✓ 2 tbsp chopped basil
- ✓ 6 black olives
- ❖ Divide the dough into 2. Roll out the crusts into circles and place on a lined baking sheet. Bake for 10 minutes. Add the cheddar cheese, marinara, eggplant, tomato and basil. Return to oven and bake for 10 minutes. Serve with olives.

Nutrition: Calories 510; Net Carbs 3.7g; Fat 39g; Protein 31g

46) Eggplant and Goat Cheese Pizza

Preparation Time: 45 minutes

Servings: 4

Ingredients:

- ✓ 4 tbsp olive oil
- ✓ 2 eggplants, sliced lengthwise
- ✓ 1 cup tomato sauce
- ✓ 2 garlic cloves, minced
- ✓ 1 red onion, sliced
- ✓ 12 ounces goat cheese, crumbled

Ingredients:

- ✓ Salt and black pepper to taste
- ✓ ½ tsp cinnamon powder
- ✓ 1 cup mozzarella cheese, shredded
- ✓ 2 tbsp oregano, chopped

Directions:

- ❖ Line a baking sheet with baking paper. Arrange eggplant slices on baking sheet and drizzle with a little olive oil. Bake for 20 minutes at 390 F. Heat the remaining olive oil in a skillet and sauté the garlic and onion for 3 minutes.

- ❖ Add goat cheese and tomato sauce and season with salt and pepper. Simmer for 10 minutes. Remove eggplant from oven and spread cheese sauce on top. Sprinkle with mozzarella cheese and oregano. Bake for 10 minutes more until cheese melts. Cut into slices and serve.

Nutrition: Calories 557; Net Carbs 8.3g; Fat 44g; Protein 33g

47) Mushroom and broccoli pizza

Preparation Time: 25 minutes

Servings: 4

Ingredients:

- ✓ ½ cup almond flour
- ✓ ¼ tsp salt
- ✓ 2 tbsp ground psyllium husk
- ✓ 2 tbsp olive oil
- ✓ 1 cup fresh sliced mushrooms
- ✓ 1 white onion, thinly sliced

Ingredients:

- ✓ 3 cups broccoli florets
- ✓ 2 cloves garlic, minced
- ✓ ½ cup unsweetened pizza sauce
- ✓ 4 tomatoes, sliced
- ✓ 1 ½ cups mozzarella cheese, grated
- ✓ ⅓ cup grated Parmesan cheese
- ❖ Heat the remaining olive oil in a skillet and sauté mushrooms, onion, garlic and broccoli for 5 minutes. Spread the pizza sauce over the crust and top with the broccoli mixture, tomato, mozzarella and Parmesan. Bake for 5 minutes. Serve in slices.

Directions:

- ❖ Preheat oven to 390 F. Line a baking sheet with parchment paper. In a bowl, mix almond flour, salt, psyllium powder, 1 tbsp olive oil and 1 cup warm water until a dough forms. Spread the dough onto the pizza pan and bake for 10 minutes.

Nutrition: Calories 180; Net carbs 3.6g; Fat 9g; Protein 17g

48) Tofu radish bowls

Preparation Time: 35 minutes

Servings: 4

Ingredients:
- ✓ ¼ cup baby mushrooms, chopped
- ✓ 2 yellow peppers, chopped
- ✓ 1 block of tofu (14 oz), cubed
- ✓ 1 tbsp + 1 tbsp olive oil
- ✓ 1 ½ cups shredded radishes

Directions:
- ❖ Heat 1 tbsp olive oil in a skillet and add tofu, radishes, onions, mushrooms and peppers; cook for 10 minutes. Divide among 4 bowls. Heat the remaining oil in the skillet, crack an egg into the pan and cook until the white sets but the yolk is quite runny.

Ingredients:
- ✓ ½ cup chopped white onions
- ✓ 4 eggs
- ✓ 1/3 cup tomato sauce
- ✓ A handful of chopped parsley
- ✓ 1 avocado, and chopped
- ❖ Transfer to the top of a bowl of tofu hash and make the remaining eggs. Top the bowls with the tomato sauce, parsley and avocado. Serve.

Nutrition: Calories 353; Net Carbs 5.9g, Fat 25g, Protein 19g

49) Tomato & Mozzarella Caprese Bake

Preparation Time: 25 minutes

Servings: 4

Ingredients:
- ✓ 4 tbsp olive oil
- ✓ 4 tomatoes, sliced
- ✓ 1 cup fresh mozzarella, sliced

Directions:
- ❖ In a baking dish, arrange the tomatoes and mozzarella slices. In a bowl, mix the pesto, mayonnaise and half of the Parmesan cheese; stir to combine.

Ingredients:
- ✓ 2 tbsp basil pesto
- ✓ 1 cup mayonnaise
- ✓ 2 ounces Parmesan cheese, grated
- ❖ Spread this mixture over the tomatoes and mozzarella and top with the remaining Parmesan cheese. Bake for 20 minutes at 360 F. Remove, let cool slightly and slice to serve.

Nutrition: Calories 420; Net Carbs 4.9g; Fat 36g; Protein 17g

50) Cookies with heart of pistachio

Preparation Time: 30 min + cooling time

Servings: 4

Ingredients:
- ✓ 1 cup butter, softened
- ✓ 2/3 cup sugar swerve
- ✓ 1 large egg, beaten
- ✓ 2 tsp pistachio extract

Directions:
- ❖ Add the butter and swerve sugar to a bowl and beat until smooth and creamy. Beat in the egg until combined. Stir in the pistachio extract and almond flour until a smooth dough forms. Wrap the dough in plastic wrap and chill for 10 minutes. Preheat oven to 350 F. Lightly dust a cutting board with almond flour. Unroll the dough and roll it out to a thickness of 2 inches.

Ingredients:
- ✓ 2 cups almond flour
- ✓ ½ cup dark chocolate
- ✓ 2 tbsp chopped pistachios

- ❖ Cut out as many cookies as you can get, while rolling back the scraps to make more cookies. Place the cookies on the baking sheet lined with parchment paper and bake for 15 minutes. Transfer to a wire rack to cool completely. Melt the dark chocolate in the microwave. Dip one side of each cookie into the melted chocolate. Garnish chocolate side with pistachios and let cool on a wire rack. Serve.

Nutrition: Calories 470; Net carbs 3.4g, fat 45g, protein 6.2g

51) Avocado and tomato burritos

Preparation Time: 10 minutes

Servings: 4

Ingredients:
- ✓ 2 cups cauli rice
- ✓ 6 low carb tortillas
- ✓ 2 cups sour cream sauce

Ingredients:
- ✓ 1 ½ cups herbed tomato sauce
- ✓ 2 avocados, peeled, pitted and sliced

Directions:
- ❖ Pour cauli rice into a bowl, sprinkle with a little water, and microwave for 2 minutes to soften. On the tortillas, spread the sour cream and spread the salsa on top.

- ❖ Top with the cauli rice and spread the avocado evenly on top. Fold and tuck the burritos and cut in half. Serve.

Nutrition: Calories 303, Fat 25g, Net Carbs 6g, Protein 8g

52) Creamy cucumber and avocado soup

Preparation Time: 15 minutes

Servings: 4

Ingredients:
- ✓ 4 large cucumbers, seeded and cut into pieces
- ✓ 1 large avocado, peeled and cut in half
- ✓ Salt and black pepper to taste
- ✓ 1 tbsp fresh cilantro, chopped
- ✓ 3 tbsp olive oil

Ingredients:
- ✓ 2 limes, squeezed
- ✓ 2 tbsp minced garlic
- ✓ 2 tomatoes, chopped
- ✓ 1 avocado, chopped for garnish

Directions:
- ❖ Pour cucumbers, avocado halves, salt, black pepper, olive oil, lime juice, cilantro, 2 cups water and garlic into food processor. Puree the ingredients for 2 minutes or until smooth.

- ❖ Pour mixture into a bowl and top with avocado and chopped tomatoes. Serve cold with zero carb bread.

Nutrition: Calories 170, Fat 7.4g, Net Carbs 4.1g, Protein 3.7g

53) Cauliflower "couscous" with lemon and Halloumi

Preparation Time: 5 minutes

Servings: 4

Ingredients:
- ✓ 4 ounces of halloumi, sliced
- ✓ 2 tbsp olive oil
- ✓ 1 head of cauliflower, cut into florets
- ✓ ¼ cup chopped cilantro

Ingredients:
- ✓ ¼ cup chopped parsley
- ✓ ¼ cup chopped mint
- ✓ ½ lemon, squeezed
- ✓ Salt and black pepper to taste
- ✓ 1 avocado, sliced for garnish

Directions:
- ❖ Heat the olive oil in a skillet over medium heat. Add halloumi and fry for 2 minutes on each side until golden brown; set aside. Pour the cauli florets into a food processor and pulse until it crumbles and resembles couscous. Transfer to a bowl and steam in the microwave for 2 minutes.

- ❖ Remove the bowl from the microwave and allow the cauli to cool. Add the cilantro, parsley, mint, lemon juice, salt and pepper. Top the couscous with avocado slices and serve with grilled halloumi and vegetable sauce.

Nutrition: Calories 185, Fat 15.6g, Net Carbs 2.1g, Protein 12g

54) Zucchini lasagna with ricotta cheese and spinach

Preparation Time: 50 minutes

Servings: 4

Ingredients:
- ✓ 2 zucchini, sliced
- ✓ Salt and black pepper to taste
- ✓ 2 cups ricotta cheese

Ingredients:
- ✓ 2 cups shredded mozzarella cheese
- ✓ 3 cups tomato sauce
- ✓ 1 cup spinach
- ❖ Repeat the layering process two more times to run out of ingredients, finally making sure to layer with the last ¼ cup of cheese mixture.
- ❖ Grease one end of the aluminum foil with cooking spray and cover the baking sheet with the foil. Bake for 35 minutes, remove the foil and bake further for 5-10 minutes or until the cheese has a nice golden brown color. Remove dish, let rest for 5 minutes, make lasagna slices and serve warm.

Directions:
- ❖ Preheat oven to 370°F. Place zucchini slices in a colander and sprinkle with salt. Let stand and drain liquid for 5 minutes and pat dry with paper towels. Mix the ricotta, mozzarella, salt and black pepper to combine evenly and spread ¼ cup of the mixture over the bottom of the baking dish.
- ❖ Arrange ⅓ of the zucchini slices on top, spread 1 cup of the tomato sauce, and scatter ⅓ cup of the spinach on top.

55) Briam with tomato sauce

Preparation Time: 40 minutes

Servings: 4

Ingredients:
- ✓ 3 tbsp olive oil
- ✓ 1 large eggplant, halved and sliced
- ✓ 1 large onion, thinly sliced
- ✓ 3 garlic cloves, sliced
- ✓ 2 tomatoes, diced
- ✓ 1 rutabaga, diced

Ingredients:
- ✓ 1 cup unsweetened tomato sauce
- ✓ 4 zucchini, sliced
- ✓ ¼ cup water
- ✓ Salt and black pepper to taste
- ✓ ¼ tsp dried oregano
- ✓ 2 tbsp fresh parsley, chopped
- ❖ Sauté the onion and garlic in the oil for 3 minutes. Remove to a bowl. Add the tomatoes, rutabaga, tomato sauce and water and mix well. Stir in salt, pepper, oregano and parsley. Pour the mixture over the eggplant and zucchini. Place the dish in the oven and bake for 25-30 minutes. Serve the briam hot.

Directions:
- ❖ Preheat oven to 400°F. Heat the olive oil in a skillet over medium heat and fry the eggplant and zucchini slices for 6 minutes until golden brown. Remove them to a casserole dish and arrange them in a single layer.

Nutrition: Calories Calories 365, Fat 12g, Net Carbohydrates 12.5g, Protein 11.3g

56) Creamy vegetable stew

Preparation Time: 25 minutes

Servings: 4

Ingredients:
- ✓ 2 tbsp ghee
- ✓ 1 tbsp onion and garlic puree
- ✓ 2 medium carrots, shredded
- ✓ 1 head of cauliflower, cut into florets

Directions:
- ❖ Melt ghee in a saucepan over medium heat and sauté onion and garlic puree to be fragrant, 2 minutes. Stir in carrots, cauliflower and green beans for 5 minutes. Season with salt and black pepper.

Ingredients:
- ✓ 2 cups green beans, cut in half
- ✓ Salt and black pepper to taste
- ✓ 1 cup water
- ✓ 1 ½ cups heavy cream
- ❖ Pour in water, stir again and cook over low heat for 15 minutes. Stir in the heavy cream to incorporate and turn off the heat. Serve the stew with almond flour bread.

Nutrition: Calories 310, fat 26.4g, net carbs 6g, protein 8g

57) Tempeh kabobs with vegetables

Preparation Time: 30 minutes + cooling time

Servings: 4

Ingredients:
- ✓ 2 tbsp ghee
- ✓ 1 tbsp onion and garlic puree
- ✓ 2 medium carrots, shredded
- ✓ 1 head of cauliflower, cut into florets

Directions:
- ❖ Melt ghee in a saucepan over medium heat and sauté onion and garlic puree to be fragrant, 2 minutes. Stir in carrots, cauliflower and green beans for 5 minutes. Season with salt and black pepper.

Ingredients:
- ✓ 2 cups green beans, cut in half
- ✓ Salt and black pepper to taste
- ✓ 1 cup water
- ✓ 1 ½ cups heavy cream
- ❖ Pour in water, stir again and cook over low heat for 15 minutes. Stir in the heavy cream to incorporate and turn off the heat. Serve the stew with almond flour bread.

Nutrition: Calories Calories 228, Fat 15g, Net Carbohydrates 3.6g, Protein 13.2g

58) Tempeh kabobs with vegetables

Preparation Time: 30 minutes + cooling time

Servings: 4

Ingredients:
- ✓ 1 yellow bell pepper, cut into pieces
- ✓ 10 ounces tempeh, cut into pieces
- ✓ 1 red onion, cut into pieces

Directions:
- ❖ Bring the 1 ½ cups of water to a boil in a pot over medium heat, and once it's cooked, turn off the heat and add the tempeh. Cover the pot and allow the tempeh to steam for 5 minutes to remove the bitterness. Drain. Pour barbecue sauce into a bowl, add tempeh and coat with sauce. Refrigerate for 2 hours.

Ingredients:
- ✓ 1 red bell bell pepper, cut into pieces
- ✓ 2 tbsp olive oil
- ✓ 1 cup unsweetened barbecue sauce
- ❖ Preheat grill to 350°F. Thread the tempeh, yellow bell pepper, red bell pepper and onion onto skewers. Brush the grill grate with olive oil, place the skewers on and brush with the barbecue sauce. Cook skewers for 3 minutes on each side, rotating and brushing with more barbecue sauce. Serve.

Nutrition: Calories Calories 228, Fat 15g, Net Carbohydrates 3.6g, Protein 13.2g

59) Cauliflower and Gouda Cheese Casserole

Preparation Time: 25 minutes

Servings: 4

Ingredients:

- ✓ 2 heads of cauliflower, cut into florets
- ✓ 2 tbsp olive oil
- ✓ 2 tbsp melted butter
- ✓ 1 white onion, chopped

Directions:

- ❖ Preheat oven to 350°F. Place cauli florets in a large microwave-safe bowl. Sprinkle with a little water and steam in the microwave for 4 to 5 minutes. Heat the olive oil in a saucepan over medium heat and sauté the onion for 3 minutes. Add the cauliflower, season with salt and pepper and stir in the almond milk.

Ingredients:

- ✓ Salt and black pepper to taste
- ✓ ¼ cup almond milk
- ✓ ½ cup almond flour
- ✓ 1 ½ cups gouda cheese, grated
- ❖ Cook over low heat for 3 minutes. Mix the melted butter with the almond flour. Stir in the cauliflower and half of the cheese. Sprinkle the top with the remaining cheese and bake for 10 minutes until the cheese is melted and golden brown on top. Plate the oven and serve with the salad.

Nutrition: Calories 215, Fat 15g, Net Carbs 4g, Protein 12g

60) Roasted Asparagus with Spicy Eggplant Sauce

Preparation Time: 35 minutes

Servings: 6

Ingredients:

- ✓ 1 ½ pounds asparagus, chopped
- ✓ ¼ cup + 2 tbsp olive oil
- ✓ ½ tsp paprika
- ✓ Eggplant Sauce
- ✓ 1 pound of eggplant
- ✓ ½ cup shallots, chopped

Directions:

- ❖ Preheat oven to 390°F. Line a parchment paper on a baking sheet. Add the asparagus. Season with 2 tbsp olive oil, paprika, black pepper and salt. Roast until cooked through, 9 minutes. Remove.
- ❖ Place the eggplant on a cookie sheet lined baking sheet. Bake in the oven for about 20 minutes.

Ingredients:

- ✓ 2 cloves garlic, minced
- ✓ 1 tbsp fresh lemon juice
- ✓ ½ tsp chili pepper
- ✓ Salt and black pepper to taste
- ✓ ¼ cup fresh cilantro, chopped

- ❖ Allow eggplant to cool. Peel them and discard the stems. Heat the remaining olive oil in a skillet over medium heat and add the garlic and shallots. Sauté for 3 minutes until tender.
- ❖ In a food processor, put together the black pepper, roasted eggplant, salt, lemon juice, shallot mixture, and red pepper. Add the cilantro and serve alongside the roasted asparagus spears.

Nutrition: Calories 149; Fat: 12.1g, Net Carbohydrates: 9g, Protein: 3.6g

61) Cook the squash

Preparation Time: 45 minutes

Servings: 6

Ingredients:

- ✓ 3 large pumpkins, peeled and sliced
- ✓ 1 cup almond flour
- ✓ 1 cup grated mozzarella cheese

Directions:

- ❖ Preheat oven to 350°F. Arrange the squash slices in a baking dish and drizzle with olive oil.

Ingredients:

- ✓ 3 tbsp olive oil
- ✓ ½ cup fresh parsley, chopped

- ❖ Bake for 35 minutes. Mix almond flour, mozzarella cheese and parsley and pour over squash. Return to oven and bake for another 5 minutes until top is golden brown. Serve warm.

Nutrition: Calories 125, Fat 4.8g, Net Carbs 5.7g, Protein 2.7g

62) Cremini Mushroom Stroganoff

Preparation Time: 25 minutes

Servings: 4

Ingredients:

- ✓ 3 tbsp butter
- ✓ 1 white onion, chopped
- ✓ 4 cups cremini mushrooms, diced

Directions:

- ❖ Melt the butter in a saucepan over medium heat and sauté the onion for 3 minutes until soft. Add the mushrooms and cook until tender, about 5 minutes. Add 2 cups of water and bring to a boil.

Ingredients:

- ✓ ½ cup heavy cream
- ✓ ½ cup Parmesan cheese, grated
- ✓ 1 ½ tbsp dried mixed herbs
- ❖ Cook for 10-15 minutes until the water reduces slightly. Pour in the heavy cream and Parmesan cheese. Stir to dissolve the cheese. Add the dried herbs and season. Simmer for 5 minutes. Serve hot.

Nutrition: Calories 284, Fat 28g, Net Carbs 1.5g, Protein 8g

63) Portobello Mushroom Burger

Preparation Time: 15 minutes

Servings: 4

Ingredients:

- ✓ 8 large portobello mushroom caps
- ✓ 1 minced garlic clove
- ✓ ½ cup of mayonnaise
- ✓ ½ tsp salt
- ✓ 4 tbsp olive oil
- ✓ ½ cup roasted red peppers, sliced

Directions:

- ❖ Preheat a grill over medium-high heat. In a bowl, crush the garlic with the salt using the back of a spoon. Stir in half the oil and brush the mushrooms and halloumi cheese with the mixture.
- ❖ Place the "sandwiches" on the skillet and grill them on both sides for 8 minutes until tender.

Ingredients:

- ✓ 2 medium tomatoes, chopped
- ✓ 4 halloumi slices, half-inch thick
- ✓ 1 tbsp red wine vinegar
- ✓ 2 tbsp Kalamata olives, chopped
- ✓ ½ tsp dried oregano
- ✓ 2 cups spinach
- ❖ Add the halloumi cheese slices to the grill. Cook for 2 minutes per side or until golden brown marks appear on the grill.
- ❖ In a bowl, mix red peppers, tomatoes, olives, vinegar, oregano, spinach and remaining olive oil; toss to coat. Spread mayonnaise on 4 mushroom "sandwiches", top with a slice of halloumi, a scoop of greens and top with remaining mushrooms. Serve and enjoy!

Nutrition: Calories 339, Fat 29.4g, Net Carbs 3.5g, Protein 10g

64) Sriracha tofu with yogurt sauce

Preparation Time: 40 minutes

Ingredients:
- ✓ 12 ounces tofu, pressed and sliced
- ✓ 1 cup green onions, chopped
- ✓ 1 clove garlic, minced
- ✓ 2 tbsp vinegar
- ✓ 1 tbsp sriracha sauce
- ✓ 2 tbsp olive oil

Directions:
- ❖ Place the tofu slices, garlic, sriracha sauce, vinegar and green onions in a bowl. Let stand for 30 minutes. Place a nonstick skillet over medium heat and add oil to heat. Cook the tofu for 5 minutes until golden brown.

Nutrition: Calories 351; Fat: 25.9g, Net Carbohydrates: 8.1g, Protein: 17.5g

Servings: 4

Ingredients:
- ✓ Yogurt Sauce
- ✓ 2 cloves garlic, crushed
- ✓ 2 tbsp fresh lemon juice
- ✓ Salt and black pepper to taste
- ✓ 1 tsp fresh dill
- ✓ 1 cup Greek yogurt
- ✓ 1 cucumber, shredded
- ❖ To make the sauce: In a bowl, mix garlic, salt, yogurt, black pepper, lemon juice and dill. Add shredded cucumber while stirring to combine. Serve tofu with a spoonful of yogurt sauce.

65) Jalapeño and Vegetable Stew

Preparation Time: 40 minutes

Ingredients:
- ✓ 2 tbsp butter
- ✓ 1 cup leeks, chopped
- ✓ 1 clove garlic, minced
- ✓ ½ cup celery stalks, chopped
- ✓ ½ cup carrots, chopped
- ✓ 1 green bell bell pepper, chopped
- ✓ 1 jalapeño bell pepper, chopped
- ✓ 1 zucchini, chopped

Directions:
- ❖ Melt the butter in a saucepan over medium heat. Add the garlic and leeks and sauté for 3 minutes until soft and translucent. Add the celery, mushrooms, zucchini and carrots and sauté for another 5 minutes.

Nutrition: Calories 65; Fat: 2.7g, Net Carbohydrates: 9g, Protein: 2.7g

Servings: 4

Ingredients:
- ✓ 1 cup mushrooms, sliced
- ✓ 1 ½ cups vegetable broth
- ✓ 2 tomatoes, chopped
- ✓ 2 tbsp fresh parsley, chopped
- ✓ 2 bay leaves
- ✓ Salt and black pepper to taste
- ✓ 1 tbsp vinegar

- ❖ Stir in the rest of the ingredients. Season with salt and pepper. Bring to a boil and simmer for 15-20 minutes or until cooked through. Divide among individual bowls and serve hot.

66) Raspberry and turmeric panna cotta

Preparation Time: 10 minutes + cooling time

Ingredients:
- ✓ ½ tbsp unflavored vegetable gelatin powder
- ✓ 2 cups of coconut cream
- ✓ ¼ tsp vanilla extract
- ✓ 1 tsp turmeric

Directions:
- ❖ Mix the gelatin and ½ tbsp water and let it dissolve. Pour the coconut cream, vanilla extract, turmeric and erythritol into a saucepan and bring to a boil; simmer for 2 minutes. Turn off the heat. Stir in gelatin.

Nutrition: Calories 270; Net Carbs 3g; Fat 27g; Protein 4g

Servings: 6

Ingredients:
- ✓ 1 tbsp erythritol
- ✓ 1 tbsp chopped toasted pecans
- ✓ 12 fresh raspberries

- ❖ Pour into 6 glasses, cover with plastic wrap and refrigerate for 2 hours. Top with pecans and raspberries and serve.

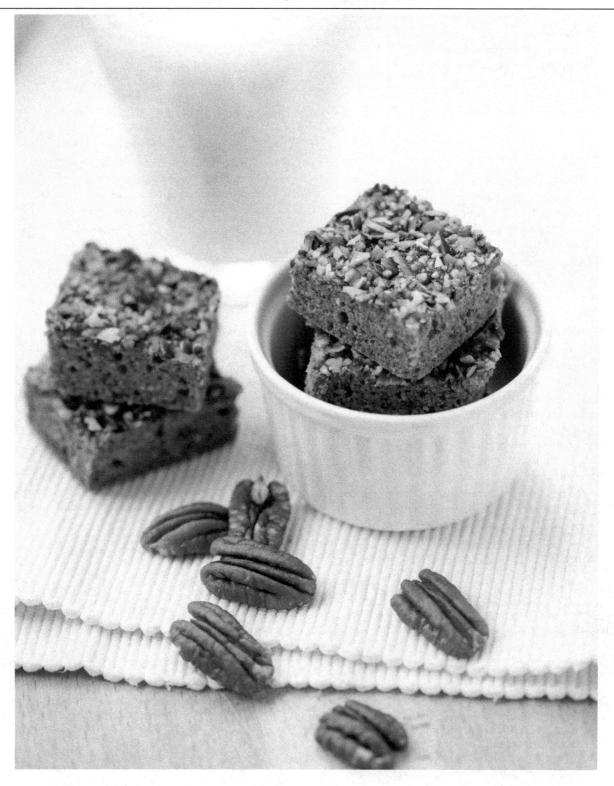

67) Chili Pepper Turnip Potatoes

Preparation Time: 50 minutes

Servings: 4

Ingredients:
- ✓ 4 large parsnips, sliced
- ✓ 3 tbsp ground pork rind

Directions:
- ❖ Preheat the oven to 425 F. Pour the parsnips into a bowl and add the pork rind. Stir and place parsnips on a baking sheet.

Ingredients:
- ✓ 3 tbsp olive oil
- ✓ ¼ tsp red pepper flakes
- ❖ Drizzle with olive oil and sprinkle with red pepper flakes. Bake until crispy, 40-45 minutes, tossing halfway through. Serve.

Nutrition: Calories 260; Net Carbs 22.6g; Fat 11g; Protein 3g

68) Buttery Radishes and Sauteed Steak

Preparation Time: 30 minutes

Servings: 4

Ingredients:
- ✓ 10 ounces tiny steak, cut into small pieces
- ✓ 3 tbsp butter
- ✓ 1½ pounds radishes, quartered

Directions:
- ❖ Melt butter in a skillet over medium heat, season meat with salt and pepper, and brown until browned on all sides, 12 minutes; transfer to a plate.

Ingredients:
- ✓ 1 clove garlic, minced
- ✓ 2 tbsp chopped fresh thyme

- ❖ Add and sauté radishes, garlic, and thyme until radishes are cooked through, 10 minutes. Plate and serve warm.

Nutrition: Calories 252; Net Carbs 0.4g; Fat 16g; Protein 21g

69) Cheddar Bacon & Celeriac Bake

Preparation Time: 50 minutes

Servings: 4

Ingredients:
- ✓ 6 slices bacon, chopped
- ✓ 3 tbsp butter
- ✓ 3 cloves garlic, minced
- ✓ 3 tbsp almond flour
- ✓ 2 cups coconut cream
- ✓ 1 cup chicken broth

Directions:
- ❖ Preheat oven to 400 F. Add bacon to a skillet and fry over medium heat until brown and crispy. Spoon onto a plate. Melt butter in the same skillet and sauté garlic for 1 minute. Add the almond flour and cook for another minute. Whisk in the coconut cream, chicken broth, salt and pepper. Cook on low heat for 5 minutes.

Ingredients:
- ✓ Salt and black pepper to taste
- ✓ 1 pound celeriac, peeled and sliced
- ✓ 2 cups shredded cheddar cheese
- ✓ ¼ cup chopped shallots

- ❖ Spread a layer of sauce in a greased casserole dish and arrange a layer of celeriac on top. Top with more sauce, top with some bacon and cheddar cheese, and scatter scallions on top. Repeat the layering process until all ingredients are used up. Bake for 35 minutes. Allow to rest for a few minutes and serve.

Nutrition: Calories 981; Net Carbs 20g; Fat 86g; Protein 28g

70) Chicken ham with mini peppers

Preparation Time: 30 minutes

Servings: 4

Ingredients:

- ✓ 12 mini green peppers, halved and seeded
- ✓ 4 slices chicken ham, chopped
- ✓ 1 tbsp chopped parsley
- ✓ 8 ounces cream cheese

Directions:

- ❖ Preheat oven to 400 F. Place peppers in a greased baking dish and set aside. In a bowl, combine the chicken ham, parsley, cream cheese, hot sauce and butter.

Ingredients:

- ✓ ½ tbsp hot sauce
- ✓ 2 tbsp melted butter
- ✓ 1 cup shredded gruyere cheese

- ❖ Spread the mixture into the peppers and sprinkle with Gruyere cheese. Bake until cheese melts, about 20 minutes. Serve.

Nutrition: Calories 408; Net carbohydrates 4g; Fat 32g; Protein 19g

71) Crispy Baked Asparagus with Cheese

Preparation Time: 40 minutes

Servings: 4

Ingredients:

- ✓ 1 cup grated Pecorino Romano cheese
- ✓ 4 slices Serrano ham, chopped
- ✓ 2 pounds asparagus, stalks chopped
- ✓ ¾ cup coconut cream

Directions:

- ❖ Preheat oven to 400 F. Arrange the asparagus on a greased baking sheet and pour the coconut cream over it. Scatter the garlic, serrano ham and pork rinds and sprinkle with the pecorino cheese, mozzarella cheese and paprika.

Ingredients:

- ✓ 3 cloves garlic, minced
- ✓ 1 cup crushed pork rind
- ✓ 1 cup grated mozzarella cheese
- ✓ ½ tsp sweet paprika
- ❖ Bake until cheese is melted and golden brown and asparagus is tender, 30 minutes.
- ❖ Serve warm.

Nutrition: Calories 361; Net Carbs 15g; Fat 21g; Protein 32g

72) Easy bacon and cheese balls

Preparation Time: 30 minutes

Servings: 4

Ingredients:

- ✓ 7 slices of bacon
- ✓ 6 ounces of cream cheese
- ✓ 6 ounces shredded Gruyere cheese

Directions:

- ❖ Place bacon in a skillet and fry over medium heat until crispy, 5 minutes. Transfer to a plate to cool and crisp. Pour the bacon grease into a bowl and stir in the cream cheese, Gruyere cheese, butter and red pepper flakes.

Ingredients:

- ✓ 2 tbsp softened butter
- ✓ ½ tsp red pepper flakes

- ❖ Place in the refrigerator to rest for 15 minutes. Remove and shape into walnut-sized balls. Roll in crumbled bacon. Plate and serve.

Nutrition: Calories 538; Net Carbs 0.5g; Fat 50g; Protein 22g

73) Cauliflower sauteed with bacon

Preparation Time: 15 minutes

Servings: 4

Ingredients:
- ✓ 1 large head of cauliflower, cut into florets
- ✓ 10 ounces bacon, chopped
- ✓ 1 clove garlic, minced

Directions:
- ❖ Pour cauliflower into boiling salted water over medium heat and cook for 5 minutes or until soft; drain and set aside.

Ingredients:
- ✓ Salt and black pepper to taste
- ✓ 2 tbsp parsley, finely chopped

- ❖ In a skillet, fry bacon until brown and crisp, 5 minutes. Add cauliflower and garlic and sauté until cauliflower is lightly browned. Season with salt and pepper. Garnish with parsley and serve.

Nutrition: Calories 243; Net Carbs 3.9g; Fat 21g; Protein 9g

74) Roasted mixed vegetables

Preparation Time: 40 minutes

Servings: 4

Ingredients:
- ✓ 2 lb butternut squash, cut into chunks
- ✓ ¼ lb pearl onions, peeled
- ✓ 2 rutabagas, cut into chunks
- ✓ 1 lb brussels sprouts
- ✓ Salt and black pepper to taste

Directions:
- ❖ Preheat the oven to 450°F. Pour the squash, pearl onions, rutabaga, garlic cloves, and Brussels sprouts into a bowl. Season with salt, black pepper, and olive oil and toss to combine.

Ingredients:
- ✓ 1 sprig rosemary, chopped
- ✓ 1 sprig thyme, chopped
- ✓ 4 garlic cloves, peeled only
- ✓ 3 tbsp olive oil

- ❖ Pour the mixture onto a baking sheet and sprinkle with the chopped thyme and rosemary. Roast the vegetables for 15-20 minutes. Once ready, remove and place in a serving bowl. Serve with baked chicken thighs.

Nutrition: Calories 65, fat 3g, net carbs 8g, protein 3g

75) Green bean chips with cheese

Preparation Time: 30 minutes

Servings: 6

Ingredients:
- ✓ ¼ cup Pecorino cheese, grated
- ✓ ¼ cup pork rind crumbs
- ✓ 1 tsp garlic powder

Directions:
- ❖ Preheat oven to 425°F and line a baking sheet with aluminum foil. Mix the cheese, pork rind, garlic powder, salt and black pepper in a bowl. Beat the eggs in another bowl.

Ingredients:
- ✓ Salt and black pepper to taste
- ✓ 2 eggs
- ✓ 1 pound green beans, stringless
- ❖ Dip the green beans in the eggs, then in the cheese mixture and arrange evenly on the baking sheet. Lightly grease with cooking spray and bake for 15 minutes to crisp. Transfer to a wire rack to cool before serving. Serve with a sugar-free tomato sauce.

Nutrition: Calories 210, Fat 19g, Net Carbs 3g, Protein 5g

76) Jalapeño Poppers Wrapped in Bacon

Preparation Time: 30 minutes

Servings: 6

Ingredients:

- ✓ 12 jalapeno peppers
- ✓ ¼ cup shredded Colby cheese

Directions:

- ❖ Cut the jalapeno peppers in half, then remove the membrane and seeds. Combine the cheeses and stuff the bell pepper halves. Wrap each bell pepper with a strip of bacon and secure with toothpicks.

Ingredients:

- ✓ 6 ounces cream cheese, softened
- ✓ 6 slices of bacon, cut in half
- ❖ Place the stuffed peppers on a baking sheet lined with aluminum foil. Bake at 350°F for 25 minutes until the bacon is golden brown and crispy and the cheese is golden brown on top. Remove to a paper towel-lined plate to absorb the grease, arrange on a serving platter and serve warm.

Nutrition: Calories 206, Fat 17g, Net Carbs 0g, Protein 14g

77) Garlic Cheddar Cookies

Preparation Time: 20 minutes

Servings: 4

Ingredients:

- ✓ ⅓ cup almond flour
- ✓ 2 tsp garlic powder
- ✓ Salt to taste
- ✓ 1 tsp baking powder

Directions:

- ❖ Preheat oven to 350°F. Mix the almond flour, garlic powder, salt, baking powder and cheddar in a bowl. In a separate bowl, beat the eggs, butter and Greek yogurt and then pour them into the dry ingredients.

Ingredients:

- ✓ 5 eggs
- ✓ ⅓ cup melted butter
- ✓ 1 ¼ cups sharp cheddar cheese, grated
- ✓ ⅓ cup Greek yogurt
- ❖ Mix well until a dough-like consistency has formed. Scoop half a tbsp of batter onto a greased baking sheet with 2-inch intervals between batters. Bake for 12 minutes to golden brown. Serve cooled.

Nutrition: Calories 153, Fat 14.2g, Net Carbs 1.4g, Protein 5.4g

78) Herb cheese sticks

Preparation Time: 15 minutes

Servings: 4

Ingredients:

- ✓ 1 cup pork rind, crushed
- ✓ 1 tbsp Italian herb blend

Directions:

- ❖ Preheat oven to 350°F. Line a baking sheet with parchment paper. Combine the pork rind and herb mix in a bowl to be evenly mixed and beat the egg in another bowl. Coat the cheese sticks in the egg.

Ingredients:

- ✓ 1 egg
- ✓ 1 pound Swiss cheese, cut into sticks
- ❖ Then, generously dip in the pork rind mixture. Arrange on the baking sheet. Bake for 4 to 5 minutes, remove later, let cool for 2 minutes and serve with marinara sauce.

Nutrition: Calories 188, Fat 17.3g, Net Carbs 0g, Protein 8g

79) Mozzarella and Prosciutto Bands

Preparation Time: 15 minutes

Servings: 6

Ingredients:

- ✓ 6 thin slices of prosciutto
- ✓ 18 basil leaves

Directions:

- ❖ Cut the prosciutto slices into three strips each. Place the basil leaves at the end of each strip. Add a scoop of cherry mozzarella.

Ingredients:

- ✓ 18 mozzarella cherry balls
- ✓ 2 tbsp of extra virgin olive oil
- ❖ Wrap the mozzarella in the prosciutto. Secure with toothpicks. Arrange on a serving platter, drizzle with olive oil and serve.

Nutrition: Calories 163, Fat: 12g, Net Carbohydrates: 0.1g, Protein: 13g

80) Avocado and Walnut Croutons

Preparation Time: 15 minutes

Servings: 4

Ingredients:

- ✓ 8 slices of zero carb bread
- ✓ 4 sheets of nori
- ✓ 1 avocado, pitted and chopped
- ✓ ⅓ tsp salt

Directions:

- ❖ In a bowl, mash the avocado with a fork. Add the salt and lemon juice and toss to combine. Place the bread slices on a baking sheet and toast them under the broiler for 3-4 minutes until golden brown.

Ingredients:

- ✓ 1 tsp lemon juice
- ✓ 1 ½ tbsp coconut oil
- ✓ ⅓ cup walnuts, chopped
- ✓ 1 tbsp poppy seeds
- ❖ Remove them and brush them with the coconut oil and spread the avocado puree on top. Garnish with the poppy seeds and walnuts, serve.

Nutrition: Calories 195, Fat 12.2g, Net Carbs 2.8g, Protein 13.7g

81) Parmesan Biscuits

Preparation Time: 25 minutes

Servings: 6

Ingredients:

- ✓ 1 ⅓ cups coconut flour
- ✓ 1 ¼ cups grated Parmesan cheese
- ✓ Salt and black pepper to taste
- ✓ 1 tsp garlic powder

Directions:

- ❖ Preheat oven to 350°F. Mix the coconut flour, Parmesan cheese, salt, pepper, garlic powder and paprika in a bowl. Add the butter and mix well. Add the heavy cream and mix again until a smooth, thick mixture forms. Add 1 to 2 tbsp of water at this point if it is too thick.

Ingredients:

- ✓ ⅓ cup butter, softened
- ✓ ⅓ tsp sweet paprika
- ✓ ⅓ cup heavy cream
- ✓ ⅓ tsp cumin seeds
- ❖ Place the dough on a cutting board and cover with plastic wrap. Use a rolling pin to roll out the dough into a light rectangle. Cut cookie squares from the dough and place them on a baking sheet without overlapping. Sprinkle with cumin seeds. Bake for 20 minutes. Serve chilled.

Nutrition: Calories 115, Fat 3g, Net Carbs 0.7g, Protein 5g

82) Spiced stuffed eggs with herbs

Preparation Time: 30 minutes

Servings: 4

Ingredients:

- ✓ 12 large eggs
- ✓ 6 tbsp of mayonnaise
- ✓ Salt and pepper to taste
- ✓ 1 tsp mixed dried herbs
- ✓ ½ tsp Worcestershire sauce

Ingredients:

- ✓ ¼ tsp Dijon mustard
- ✓ ½ tsp sweet paprika
- ✓ 2 tbsp fresh parsley, chopped

Directions:

- ❖ Pour salted water into a saucepan and bring to a boil over high heat. Add eggs and cook for 10 minutes. Remove to an ice bath and allow to cool. Peel and cut in half lengthwise and place yolks in a bowl.

- ❖ Use a fork to mash them. Add the mayonnaise, salt, chili, dried herbs, Worcestershire sauce, mustard and paprika. Mix until a smooth paste forms. Then, pour the mixture into a pastry bag and fill in the egg white holes. Garnish with parsley and serve immediately.

Nutrition: Calories 112, Fat 9.3g, Net Carbs 0.4g, Protein 6.7g

83) Roast green beans and mozzarella cheese with bacon

Preparation Time: 30 minutes

Servings: 4

Ingredients:

- ✓ 2 tbsp olive oil
- ✓ 1 tsp of onion powder
- ✓ 1 beaten egg

Ingredients:

- ✓ 15 ounces fresh green beans
- ✓ 5 tbsp grated mozzarella cheese
- ✓ 4 slices bacon, chopped
- ❖ Pour the mixture onto the baking sheet and bake until the green beans turn slightly brown and the cheese melts, 20 minutes. Fry the bacon in a skillet until crisp and brown. Remove green beans and divide among serving plates. Add bacon and serve.

Directions:

- ❖ Preheat oven to 350 F. Line a baking sheet with parchment paper. In a bowl, mix the olive oil, onion and garlic powder, and egg. Add the green beans and mozzarella cheese and stir to coat.

Nutrition: Calories 208; Net carbs 2.6g; Fat 19g; Protein 6g

84) Salami and cheese skewers

Preparation Time: 10 minutes + cooling time

Servings: 4

Ingredients:

- ✓ ¼ cup olive oil
- ✓ 1 tbsp plain vinegar
- ✓ 2 cloves garlic, minced
- ✓ 1 tsp dried Italian herb mixture

Ingredients:

- ✓ 4 ounces hard salami, cubed
- ✓ ¼ cup pitted Kalamata olives
- ✓ 12 ounces cheddar cheese, cubed
- ✓ 1 tsp chopped parsley
- ❖ Remove, drain marinade and thread a cube of salami, olive and cheese cube onto a skewer. Repeat by making more skewers with the remaining ingredients. Garnish with parsley and serve.

Directions:

- ❖ In a bowl, mix olive oil, vinegar, garlic and herb mixture. Add salami, olives and cheddar cheese. Stir until well coated. Cover bowl with plastic wrap and marinate in refrigerator for 4 hours.

Nutrition: Calories 585; Net carbs 1.8g; Fat 52g; Protein 27g

85) Baked zucchini sticks with chili and Aioli

Preparation Time: 25 minutes

Servings: 4

Ingredients:

✓ ¼ cup Pecorino Romano cheese, shredded
✓ ¼ cup pork rind crumbs
✓ 1 tsp sweet paprika
✓ Salt and chili pepper to taste
✓ 1 cup mayonnaise

Directions:

❖ Preheat oven to 425 F. Line a baking sheet with aluminum foil. In a bowl, mix the pork rinds, paprika, pecorino romano, salt and pepper. Beat the eggs in another bowl. Coat the zucchini strips in the eggs, then in the cheese mixture and arrange on the baking sheet.

Nutrition: Calories 180; Net carbs 2g; Fat 14g; Protein 6g

Ingredients:

✓ Juice of half a lemon
✓ 2 cloves of garlic, minced
✓ 3 fresh eggs
✓ 2 zucchini, cut into strips

❖ Lightly grease with cooking spray and bake for 15 minutes. Combine the mayonnaise, lemon juice, and garlic in a bowl and mix gently until everything is well incorporated. Serve the strips with the aioli.

86) Cauliflower rice and bacon gratin

Preparation Time: 30 minutes   **Servings: 4**

Ingredients:

✓ 1 cup canned artichoke hearts, drained and chopped
✓ 6 slices bacon, chopped
✓ 2 cups cauliflower rice
✓ 3 cups spinach, chopped
✓ 1 clove garlic, minced
✓ 1 tbsp olive oil

Directions:

❖ Preheat oven to 350 F. Cook bacon in a skillet over medium heat until brown and crispy, 5 minutes. Spoon onto a plate. In a bowl, mix Cauli rice, artichokes, spinach, garlic, olive oil, salt, pepper, sour cream, cream cheese, bacon and half of the Parmesan cheese.

Nutrition: Calories 500; Net Carbs 5.3g; Fat 37g; Protein 28g

Ingredients:

✓ Salt and black pepper to taste
✓ ¼ cup sour cream
✓ 8 ounces cream cheese, softened
✓ ¼ cup grated Parmesan cheese
✓ 1 ½ cups grated mozzarella cheese

❖ Spread the mixture on a baking sheet and top with the remaining Parmesan and mozzarella. Bake for 15 minutes. Serve.

87) Delicious Strawberries with Bacon

Preparation Time: 30 minutes   **Servings: 4**

Ingredients:

✓ 2 tbsp powdered sugar swerve
✓ 1 cup mascarpone cheese
✓ 1/8 tsp white pepper

Directions:

❖ In a bowl, combine the mascarpone, powdered sugar and white pepper. Coat the strawberries in the mixture, wrap each strawberry in a slice of bacon, and place on an ungreased baking sheet.

Nutrition: Calories 171; Net Carbs 1.2g; Fat 11g; Protein 12g

Ingredients:

✓ 12 fresh strawberries
✓ 12 thin slices of bacon

❖ Bake at 425 F for 15-20 minutes until bacon is brown. Serve warm.

88) Creamy ham and parsnip puree

Preparation Time: 45 minutes

Servings: 4

Ingredients:

- ✓ 1 pound parsnips, diced
- ✓ 3 tbsp olive oil, divided
- ✓ 2 tsp garlic powder
- ✓ ¾ cup almond milk

Directions:

- ❖ Preheat oven to 400 F. Spread parsnips on a baking sheet and drizzle with 2 tbsp olive oil. Cover tightly with aluminum foil and bake until the parsnips are tender, 40 minutes.

Ingredients:

- ✓ 4 tbsp heavy cream
- ✓ 4 tbsp butter
- ✓ 6 slices prosciutto, chopped
- ✓ 2 tsp fresh oregano, chopped
- ❖ Remove from oven, remove foil and transfer to a bowl. Add the garlic powder, almond milk, heavy cream and butter. Using an immersion blender, blend ingredients until smooth. Add the ham and sprinkle with oregano. Serve.

Nutrition: Calories 477; Net carbs 20g; Fat 30g; Protein 10g

89) Roasted ham with radishes

Preparation Time: 30 minutes

Servings: 4

Ingredients:

- ✓ 1 pound radishes, halved
- ✓ Salt and black pepper to taste

Directions:

- ❖ Preheat oven to 375 F. Arrange radishes on a greased baking sheet.

Ingredients:

- ✓ 1 tbsp melted butter
- ✓ 3 slices ham, chopped

- ❖ Season with salt and pepper and sprinkle with butter and ham. Bake for 25 minutes. Serve warm.

Nutrition: Calories 68; Net Carbs 0.5g; Fat 4g; Protein 4g

90) Rosemary cheese chips with guacamole

Preparation Time: 20 minutes

Servings: 4

Ingredients:

- ✓ 1 tbsp rosemary, chopped
- ✓ 1 cup Grana Padano cheese, grated
- ✓ ¼ tsp sweet paprika

Directions:

- ❖ Preheat oven to 350 F. Line a baking sheet with parchment paper. Mix Grana Padano cheese, paprika, rosemary and garlic powder evenly. Spread 6-8 tsp on baking sheet, creating spaces between each pile; flatten piles. Bake for 5 minutes, cool and remove to a plate.

Ingredients:

- ✓ ¼ tsp garlic powder
- ✓ 2 avocados, pitted and mashed
- ✓ 1 tomato, chopped
- ❖ To make the guacamole, mash the avocado with a fork in a bowl, add the tomato and continue mashing until smooth; season. Serve the chips with the guacamole.

Nutrition: Calories 229; Net Carbs 2g; Fat 20g; Protein 10g

91) Ham rolls with chives and green beans

Preparation Time: 15 minutes + cooling time

Servings: 4

Ingredients:
- ✓ 8 ounces Havarti cheese, cut into 16 strips
- ✓ 16 thin slices of prosciutto, cut in half lengthwise
- ✓ 1 medium sweet red bell pepper, cut into 16 strips
- ✓ 1 ½ cups water

Directions:
- ❖ Bring water to a boil in a saucepan over medium heat. Add green beans, cover and cook for 3 minutes or until softened; drain. Melt butter in a skillet and sauté green beans for 2 minutes; transfer to a plate.

Ingredients:
- ✓ 16 fresh green beans
- ✓ 2 tbsp salted butter
- ✓ 16 whole chives

- ❖ Assemble 1 green bean, 1 strip of red bell pepper, 1 strip of cheese and wrap with a slice of ham. Tie with a chive. Repeat assembly process with remaining ingredients and refrigerate.

Nutrition: Calories 399; Net carbs 8.7g; Fat 24g; Protein 35g

92) Crunchy rutabaga puff pastries

Preparation Time: 35 minutes

Servings: 4

Ingredients:
- ✓ 1 rutabaga, peeled and diced
- ✓ 2 tbsp melted butter

Directions:
- ❖ Preheat oven to 400 F. Spread the rutabaga on a baking sheet and drizzle with butter. Bake until tender, 15 minutes. Transfer to a bowl. Allow to cool and add the goat cheese. Using a fork, mash and mix ingredients together.

Ingredients:
- ✓ ½ oz goat cheese, crumbled
- ✓ ¼ cup ground pork rinds
- ❖ Pour pork rinds onto a plate. Form 1-inch balls with the rutabaga mixture and roll them properly in the pork rind, pressing gently to adhere. Place in the same baking dish and bake for 10 minutes until golden brown. Serve.

Nutrition: Calories 129; Net carbohydrates 5.9g; Fat 8g; Protein 3g

93) Crispy Roast Bacon and Butternut Squash

Preparation Time: 30 minutes

Servings: 4

Ingredients:
- ✓ 2 butternut squash, cut into cubes
- ✓ 1 tsp turmeric powder
- ✓ ½ tsp garlic powder

Directions:
- ❖ Preheat the oven to 425 F. In a bowl, add the squash, turmeric, garlic powder, bacon and olive oil. Stir until well coated.

Ingredients:
- ✓ 8 slices of bacon, chopped
- ✓ 2 tbsp olive oil
- ✓ 1 tbsp chopped cilantro,
- ❖ Spread the mixture onto a greased baking sheet and roast for 10-15 minutes. Transfer vegetables to a bowl and garnish with cilantro to serve.

Nutrition: Calories 148; Net Carbs 6.4g; Fat 10g; Protein 6g

94) Eggs with paprika and dill

Preparation Time: 20 minutes

Servings: 4

Ingredients:
- ✓ 1 tsp dill, chopped
- ✓ 8 large eggs
- ✓ 3 cups water

Directions:
- ❖ Bring eggs to a boil in salted water and cook for 10 minutes. Transfer to an ice water bath, let cool completely and peel the shells. Cut the eggs in half lengthwise and empty the yolks into a bowl. Mash with a fork and mix with the sriracha sauce, mayonnaise and paprika until smooth.

Ingredients:
- ✓ 3 tbsp sriracha sauce
- ✓ 4 tbsp mayonnaise
- ✓ ¼ tsp sweet paprika
- ❖ Pour filling into a pastry bag and fill egg whites so they are slightly above the rim. Garnish with dill and serve.

Nutrition: Calories 195; Net carbs 1g; Fat 19g; Protein 4g

95) Plain Stuffed Eggs with Mayonnaise

Preparation Time: 30 minutes

Servings: 6

Ingredients:
- ✓ 6 eggs
- ✓ 1 tbsp tabasco verde

Directions:
- ❖ Place eggs in boiling salted water and cook for 10 minutes. Remove eggs to an ice bath and allow to cool. Peel and cut in half lengthwise.

Ingredients:
- ✓ ¼ cup mayonnaise
- ✓ 2 tbsp black olives, sliced
- ❖ Scoop the yolks into a bowl and mash them with a fork. Whisk together the tabasco, mayonnaise and crushed yolks in a bowl. Pour this mixture into the egg whites. Garnish with olives and serve.

Nutrition: Calories 178; Net carbohydrates: 5g; Fat: 17g; Protein: 6g

96) Pork rind bread with cheese

Preparation Time: 30 minutes

Servings: 4

Ingredients:
- ✓ ¼ cup grated Pecorino Romano cheese
- ✓ 8 ounces of cream cheese
- ✓ 2 cups grated mozzarella cheese
- ✓ 1 tbsp baking powder

Directions:
- ❖ Preheat oven to 375 F. Line a baking sheet with baking paper. Microwave the cream cheese and mozzarella cheese for 1 minute or until melted.

Ingredients:
- ✓ 1 cup crushed pork rind
- ✓ 3 large eggs
- ✓ 1 tbsp mixed Italian herbs

- ❖ Blend baking powder, pork rind, eggs, pecorino romano cheese and Italian mixed herbs. Spread mixture into baking dish and bake for 20 minutes until lightly brown. Let cool, slice and serve.

Nutrition: Calories 437; Net Carbs 3.2g; Fat 23g; Protein 32g

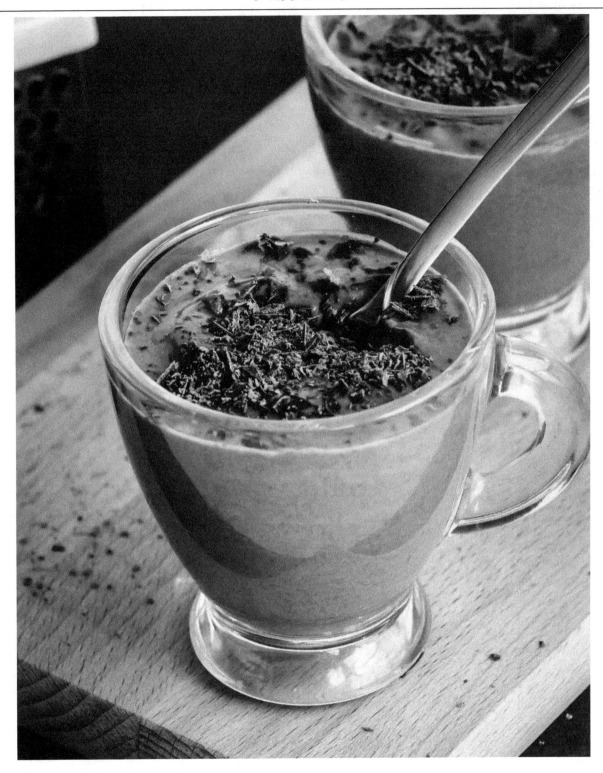

97) Orange Delight

Preparation Time: 35 minutes

Servings: 2

Ingredients:
- ✓ Juice of 2 lemons
- ✓ 6 tbsp of stevia

Ingredients:
- ✓ 1 pound of oranges, peeled and cut in half
- ✓ 1 pint of water
- ❖ Divide into jars and serve cold.

Directions:
- ❖ In Instant Pot, mix lemon juice with orange juice and orange segments, water and stevia, cover and cook over high heat for 15 minutes.

Nutrition: Calories 75 | Fat: 0g | Carbohydrates: 2g | Protein: 2g | Fiber: 0g | Sugar: 5g

98) Simple Pumpkin Pie

Preparation Time: 2 minutes

Servings: 25

Ingredients:
- ✓ 2 pounds of pumpkin, peeled and cut into pieces
- ✓ 2 eggs
- ✓ 2 cups water
- ✓ 1 cup of coconut milk
- ✓ 2 tbsp of honey

Ingredients:
- ✓ 1 tsp cinnamon powder
- ✓ ½ tsp ginger powder
- ✓ ¼ tsp. cloves, ground
- ✓ 1 tbsp arrowroot powder
- ✓ Chopped pecans
- ❖ Add the rest of the water to the Instant Pot, add the steamer basket, add ramekins inside, cover and cook on high heat for 10 minutes.
- ❖ Garnish with chopped pecans and serve.
- ❖ Enjoy!

Directions:
- ❖ Place 1 cup of water in the Instant Pot, add the steamer basket, add the pumpkin pieces, cover, cook on high heat for 4 minutes, drain, transfer to a bowl and mash.
- ❖ Add honey, milk, eggs, cinnamon, ginger and cloves, mix very well and pour into ramekins.

Nutrition: Calories 132 | Fat: 1g | Carbohydrates: 2g | Protein: 3g | Fiber: 2g | Sugar: 0g

99) Green Tea Brownies with Macadamia Nuts

Preparation Time: 28 minutes

Servings: 4

Ingredients:
- ✓ 1 tbsp green tea powder
- ✓ ¼ cup unsalted butter, melted
- ✓ 4 tbsp powdered sugar swerve
- ✓ A pinch of salt

Ingredients:
- ✓ ¼ cup coconut flour
- ✓ ½ tsp baking powder
- ✓ 1 egg
- ✓ ¼ cup chopped macadamia nuts
- ❖ Beat the mixture until the egg is incorporated. Pour the coconut flour, green tea and baking powder into a fine mesh sieve, sift into the egg bowl and stir. Add the walnuts, mix again and pour the mixture into the lined baking dish. Bake for 18 minutes, remove and dice the brownies.

Directions:
- ❖ Preheat oven to 350°F and line a square baking sheet with baking paper. Pour the melted butter into a bowl, add the sugar and salt and beat to combine. Crack the egg into the bowl.

Nutrition: Calories 248, Fat 23.1g, Net Carbs 2.2g, Protein 5.2g

100) Lychee and Coconut Lassi

Preparation Time: 30 minutes + cooling time

Servings: 4

Ingredients:
- ✓ 2 cups lychee pulp, seeded
- ✓ 2 ½ cups coconut milk
- ✓ 4 tbsp of swerve sugar
- ✓ 2 limes, peeled and squeezed

Ingredients:
- ✓ 1 ½ cups plain yogurt
- ✓ 1 lemongrass, white part only, torn off
- ✓ 2 tbsp toasted coconut flakes
- ✓ A pinch of salt
- ❖ Remove the lemongrass and pour the mixture into a smoothie machine or blender. Add the yogurt, salt, and lime juice and process the ingredients until smooth, about 60 seconds. Pour into a pitcher and refrigerate for 2 hours until cold; stir. Serve garnished with coconut shavings.

Directions:
- ❖ In a saucepan, add the lychee pulp, coconut milk, swerve sugar, lemongrass and lime zest. Stir and bring to a boil over medium heat for 2 minutes, stirring constantly. Then reduce the heat and simmer for 1 minute. Turn off the heat and let the mixture sit for 15 minutes.

Nutrition: Calories 285, Fat 26.1g, Net Carbs 1.5g, Protein 5.3g

101) Lemon Cheesecake Mousse

Preparation Time: 5 minutes + cooling time

Servings: 4

Ingredients:
- ✓ 24 ounces cream cheese, softened
- ✓ 2 cups powdered sugar swerve
- ✓ 2 lemons, squeezed and peeled

Ingredients:
- ✓ ¼ tsp salt
- ✓ 1 ¼ cups whipped cream

- ❖ Pour mousse into serving cups and refrigerate to thicken for 1 hour. Drizzle with remaining whipped cream and lightly garnish with lemon zest. Allow to rest in the refrigerator before serving.

Directions:
- ❖ Whip the cream cheese in a bowl with a hand mixer until light and fluffy. Mix in the swerve sugar, lemon juice and salt. Add 1 cup of the whipped cream to combine evenly.

Nutrition: Calories 223, fat 18g, net carbs 3g, protein 12g

102) Chocolate Mint Protein Smoothie

Preparation Time: 4 minutes

Servings: 4

Ingredients:
- ✓ 3 cups of flax milk, chilled
- ✓ 3 tbsp unsweetened cocoa powder
- ✓ 1 avocado, pitted, peeled, sliced
- ✓ 1 cup coconut milk, cooled

Ingredients:
- ✓ 3 mint leaves + more for garnish
- ✓ 3 tbsp erythritol
- ✓ 1 tbsp low-carb protein powder
- ✓ Whipping cream for garnish
- ❖ Pour into serving glasses, lightly top with whipping cream and garnish with mint leaves.

Directions:
- ❖ Combine milk, cocoa powder, avocado, coconut milk, mint leaves, erythritol and protein powder in a blender and blend for 1 minute until smooth.

Nutrition: Calories 191, Fat 14.5g, Net Carbs 4g, Protein 15g

103) Chia and blackberry pudding

Preparation Time: 10 minutes + cooling time

Servings: 2

Ingredients:

- ✓ 1 cup whole natural yogurt
- ✓ 2 tbsp sugar swerve
- ✓ 2 tbsp chia seeds

Ingredients:

- ✓ 1 cup fresh blackberries
- ✓ 1 tbsp lemon zest
- ✓ Mint leaves, to serve
- ❖ Refrigerate for 30 minutes. Divide the mixture between 2 glasses. Add a couple of blackberries, the mint and lemon zest to each. Serve.

Directions:

- ❖ In a bowl, mix the yogurt and swerve sugar. Stir in the chia seeds. Reserve 4 blackberries for garnish. Mash the remaining ones with a fork. Stir into yogurt mixture.

Nutrition: Calories 169, Fat: 10g, Net Carbs: 4.7g, Protein: 7.5g

104) Strawberry and Basil Lemonade

Preparation Time: 3 minutes

Servings: 4

Ingredients:

- ✓ 4 cups water
- ✓ 12 strawberries, leafless
- ✓ 1 cup fresh lemon juice
- ✓ ⅓ cup fresh basil

Ingredients:

- ✓ ¾ cup sugar swerve
- ✓ Crushed ice
- ✓ Halved strawberries for garnish
- ✓ Basil leaves for garnish
- ❖ The mixture should be pink, and the basil finely chopped. Adjust taste. Drop 2 strawberry halves and some basil into each glass and serve immediately.

Directions:

- ❖ Pour crushed ice into 4 serving glasses and set aside. In a pitcher, add the water, strawberries, lemon juice, basil and swerve. Turn on the blender and process the ingredients for 30 seconds.

Nutrition: Calories 66, Fat 0.1g, Net Carbs 5.8g, Protein 0.7g

105) Vanilla Chocolate Mousse

Preparation Time: 30 minutes

Servings: 4

Ingredients:

- ✓ 3 eggs
- ✓ 1 cup dark chocolate chips
- ✓ 1 cup heavy cream

Ingredients:

- ✓ 1 cup fresh strawberries, sliced
- ✓ 1 vanilla extract
- ✓ 1 tbsp sugar swerve
- ❖ Add the eggs, vanilla extract, and reserve; beat to combine. Add the cooled chocolate. Divide the mousse among four glasses, top with the strawberry slices and chill in the refrigerator for at least 30 minutes before serving.

Directions:

- ❖ Melt the chocolate in a bowl, in your microwave for one minute on high speed, and let it cool for 10 minutes.
- ❖ Meanwhile, in a medium sized bowl, whip the cream until very smooth.

Nutrition: Calories 370, Fat: 25g, Net Carbs: 3.7g, Protein: 7.6g

106) Cranberry chocolate barks

Preparation Time: 5 minutes + cooling time

Servings: 6

Ingredients:
- ✓ 10 ounces unsweetened dark chocolate, chopped
- ✓ ½ cup erythritol
- ✓ ⅓ cup dried blueberries, chopped

Directions:
- ❖ Line a baking sheet with parchment paper. Pour the chocolate and erythritol into a bowl, and melt in the microwave for 25 seconds, stirring three times until completely melted.

Ingredients:
- ✓ ⅓ cup toasted walnuts, chopped
- ✓ ¼ tbsp darkened race
- ✓ ¼ tsp salt
- ❖ Stir in blueberries, dark rum, walnuts and salt, reserving some blueberries and walnuts for garnish.
- ❖ Pour the mixture onto the baking sheet and spread it out. Sprinkle with the remaining blueberries and walnuts. Refrigerate for 2 hours to rest. Break into bite-size pieces to serve.

Nutrition: Calories 225, Fat 21g, Net Carbs 3g, Protein 6g

107) Chocolate Cheesecake Bites

Preparation Time: 4 minutes + cooling time

Servings: 12

Ingredients:
- ✓ 10 ounces unsweetened dark chocolate chips
- ✓ ½ half and half

Directions:
- ❖ In a saucepan, melt chocolate with half and half over low heat for 1 minute. Turn off the heat. In a bowl, beat cream cheese, swerve sugar and vanilla extract with a hand mixer until smooth.

Ingredients:
- ✓ 20 ounces cream cheese, softened
- ✓ 1 tsp vanilla extract
- ❖ Stir into chocolate mixture. Spoon into silicone muffin tins and freeze for 4 hours until firm.

Nutrition: Calories 241, Fat 22g, Net Carbs 3.1g, Protein 5g

108) Blueberry Popsicles

Preparation Time: 5 minutes + cooling time

Servings: 6

Ingredients:
- ✓ 3 cups blueberries
- ✓ ½ tbsp lemon juice

Directions:
- ❖ Pour blueberries, lemon juice, sugar swerve and ¼ cup water into a blender and blend on high speed for 2 minutes until smooth. Strain through a sieve into a bowl, discarding solids.

Ingredients:
- ✓ ¼ cup of reserved sugar

- ❖ Stir in more water if too thick. Divide mixture into ice pop molds, insert stick lid and freeze 4 hours to 1 week. When ready to serve, submerge in hot water and remove pops.

Nutrition: Calories 48, Fat 1.2g, Net Carbohydrates 7.9g, Protein 2.3g

109)   Special Vanilla Dessert

Preparation Time: 25 minutes

Servings: 2

Ingredients:
- ✓ 1 cup almond milk
- ✓ 4 tbsp of flax flour
- ✓ 2 tbsp of coconut flour
- ✓ 2 ½ cups water

Directions:
- ❖ In your Instant Pot, mix flax meal with flour, water, stevia, milk and espresso powder, stir, cover and cook on high heat for 10 minutes.

Ingredients:
- ✓ 2 tbsp stevia
- ✓ 1 tbsp espresso powder
- ✓ 2 tbsp vanilla extract
- ✓ Coconut cream to serve
- ❖ Add vanilla extract, mix well, set aside for 5 minutes, divide into bowls and serve with coconut cream on top.
- ❖ Enjoy!

Nutrition: Calories 182 | Fat: 2g | Carbohydrates: 3g | Protein: 4g | Fiber: 10.6g | Sugar: 1g

110)   Tasty and surprising dessert with pears

It's easy to make this tasty and unique dish

Preparation Time: 25 minutes

Servings: 2

Ingredients:
- ✓ 1 cup water
- ✓ 2 cups of pear, peeled and diced
- ✓ 2 cups of coconut milk
- ✓ 1 tbsp of ghee
- ✓ ¼ cup brown stevia

Directions:
- ❖ In a heatproof dish, mix milk with stevia, ghee, flax meal, cinnamon, raisins, pears and walnuts and stir.
- ❖ Place water in Instant Pot, add steamer basket, place heatproof dish inside, cover and cook on high heat for 6 minutes.

Ingredients:
- ✓ ½ tbsp cinnamon powder
- ✓ 4 tbsp flax meal
- ✓ ½ cup walnuts, chopped
- ✓ ½ cup raisins

- ❖ Divide this large dessert into small cups and serve cold.
- ❖ Enjoy!

Nutrition: Calories 162 | Fat: 3g | Carbohydrates: 2g | Protein: 6g | Fiber: 1g | Sugar: 1g

111)   Strawberry and Vanilla Smoothie

Preparation Time: 2 minutes

Servings: 4

Ingredients:
- ✓ 2 cups strawberries, cut in half
- ✓ 12 strawberries for garnish
- ✓ ½ cup unsweetened almond milk

Directions:
- ❖ Process strawberries, milk, vanilla extract, whipping cream and swerve in a large blender for 2 minutes; process in two batches if necessary.

Ingredients:
- ✓ 2/3 tsp vanilla extract
- ✓ ½ cup heavy whipping cream
- ✓ 2 tbsp sugar swerve
- ❖ Smoothie should be frosty. Pour into glasses, thread through straws, garnish with strawberry halves and serve.

Nutrition: Kcal 285, Fat 22.6g, Net Carbs 3.1g, Protein 16g

112)   Black Currant Iced Tea

Preparation Time: 10 minutes

Ingredients:
- ✓ ½ cup sugar-free blackcurrant extract
- ✓ 6 unflavored tea bags
- ✓ Sabre to taste

Directions:
- ❖ Pour ice cubes into a pitcher and refrigerate. Bring 2 cups of water to a boil in a saucepan over medium heat for 3 minutes and turn off the heat. Stir in the sugar to dissolve it and steep the tea bags in the water for 2 minutes. Remove the bags afterwards and allow the tea to cool.

Ingredients:
- ✓ Ice cubes for serving
- ✓ Lemon slices for garnish

- ❖ Stir in the black currant extract until well incorporated, remove the pitcher from the refrigerator and pour the mixture over the ice cubes. Let sit for 3 minutes to cool and after, pour the mixture into tall glasses. Add more ice cubes, place lemon slices on the rim of the glasses and serve the iced tea.

Nutrition: Kcal 22, Fat 0g, Net Carbs 5g, Protein 0g

113)   Cinnamon Turmeric Milk

Preparation Time: 7 minutes

Ingredients:
- ✓ 3 cups almond milk
- ✓ ⅓ tsp cinnamon powder
- ✓ 1 cup of brewed coffee

Directions:
- ❖ In a blender, add the almond milk, cinnamon powder, coffee, turmeric and erythritol. Blend the ingredients on medium speed for 45 seconds and pour the mixture into a saucepan.

Ingredients:
- ✓ ½ tsp turmeric powder
- ✓ 1 ½ tsp erythritol
- ✓ Cinnamon sticks for garnish
- ❖ Place the saucepan over low heat and heat for 5 minutes; do not boil. Continue to shake the pan to prevent boiling. Turn off the heat and serve in mugs of milk, with a cinnamon stick in each.

Nutrition: Kcal 132, Fat 12g, Net Carbohydrates 0.3g, Protein 3.9g

114)   Almond Butter Fat Bombs

Preparation Time: 3 minutes + cooling time

Ingredients:
- ✓ ½ cup almond butter
- ✓ ½ cup coconut oil

Directions:
- ❖ Melt the butter and coconut oil in the microwave for 45 seconds, stirring twice until melted and mixed properly.

Ingredients:
- ✓ 4 tbsp unsweetened cocoa powder
- ✓ ½ cup erythritol
- ❖ Stir in the cocoa powder and erythritol until fully combined. Pour into muffin molds and refrigerate for 3 hours to harden.

Nutrition: Kcal 193, Fat 18.3g, Net Carbs 2g, Protein 4g

115)   Almond Milk Hot Chocolate

Preparation Time: 7 minutes

Servings: 4

Ingredients:

- ✓ 3 cups almond milk
- ✓ 4 tbsp unsweetened cocoa powder
- ✓ 2 tbsp of swerve sugar

Directions:

- ❖ In a saucepan, add the almond milk, cocoa powder and swerve sugar. Stir the mixture until the sugar dissolves. Place the saucepan on low heat to heat for 5 minutes, without boiling.

Ingredients:

- ✓ 3 tbsp almond butter
- ✓ Finely chopped almonds for garnish

- ❖ Stir the mixture occasionally. Turn off the heat and stir in the almond butter to be incorporated. Pour hot chocolate into mugs and sprinkle with chopped almonds. Serve warm.

Nutrition: Kcal 225, Fat 21.5g, Net Carbs 0.6g, Protein 4.5g

116)   Raspberry Flaxseed Dessert

Preparation Time: 5 minutes

Servings: 4

Ingredients:

- ✓ 2 cups raspberries, reserving some for garnish
- ✓ 3 cups unsweetened vanilla almond milk
- ✓ 1 cup heavy cream
- ✓ ½ cup chia seeds

Directions:

- ❖ In a medium bowl, mash raspberries with a fork until pureed. Pour in the almond milk, heavy cream, chia seeds and liquid stevia. Stir and refrigerate the pudding overnight.

Ingredients:

- ✓ ½ cup flax seeds, ground
- ✓ 4 tbsp liquid stevia
- ✓ Chopped mixed nuts for garnish

- ❖ Pour pudding into serving glasses, top with raspberries, mixed nuts and serve.

Nutrition: Kcal 390, Fat 33.5g, Net Carbs 3g, Protein 13g

117)   Merry Berry

Preparation Time: 6 minutes

Servings: 4

Ingredients:

- ✓ 1 cup strawberries + extra for garnish
- ✓ 1 ½ cups blackberries
- ✓ 1 cup blueberries

Directions:

- ❖ For extra strawberries for garnish, make a single deep cut on their sides; set aside. Add blackberries, strawberries, blueberries, beets and ice cubes to smoothie maker.

Ingredients:

- ✓ 2 small beets, peeled and chopped
- ✓ 2/3 cup ice cubes
- ✓ 1 lime, squeezed
- ❖ Blend ingredients on high speed until smooth and frothy, about 60 seconds. Add the lime juice and blend for 30 seconds more. Pour the drink into tall smoothie glasses, secure the reserved strawberries on the rim of each glass, stick a straw in and serve the drink immediately.

Nutrition: Kcal 83, Fat 3g, Net Carbs 8g, Protein 2.7g

118) Cinnamon Cookies

Preparation Time: 25 minutes

Ingredients:

- ✓ Cookies
- ✓ 2 cups almond flour
- ✓ ½ tsp baking soda
- ✓ ¾ cup sweetener
- ✓ ½ cup butter, softened

Directions:

- ❖ Preheat oven to 350°F. Combine all cookie ingredients in a bowl. Make 16 balls with the dough and flatten them with your hands. Combine the cinnamon and erythritol.

Nutrition: Kcal 134, Fat: 13g, Net Carbs: 1.5g, Protein: 3g

Ingredients:

- ✓ A pinch of salt
- ✓ Coating
- ✓ 2 tbsp erythritol sweetener
- ✓ 1 tsp cinnamon

- ❖ Dip the cookies into the cinnamon mixture and place them on a lined baking sheet. Bake for 15 minutes, until crispy.

119) Vanilla Frappuccino

Preparation Time: 6 minutes

Servings: 4

Ingredients:

- ✓ 3 cups unsweetened vanilla almond milk, chilled Unsweetened chocolate chips for garnish
- ✓ 2 tbsp sugar swerve
- ✓ 1 ½ cups heavy cream, chilled

Directions:

- ❖ Combine almond milk, swerve sugar, heavy cream, vanilla bean and xanthan gum in blender and process on high speed for 1 minute until smooth.

Nutrition: Kcal 193, Fat 14g, Net Carbs 6g, Protein 15g

Ingredients:

- ✓ 1 vanilla bean
- ✓ ¼ tsp xanthan gum

- ❖ Pour into tall shake glasses, sprinkle with chocolate chips and serve immediately.

120) Peanut Butter Pecan Ice Cream

Preparation Time: 36 minutes + cooling time

Servings: 4

Ingredients:

- ✓ ½ cup swerve confectioners sweetener
- ✓ 2 cups heavy cream
- ✓ 1 tbsp of erythritol
- ✓ ½ cup plain peanut butter

Directions:

- ❖ Heat the heavy cream with the peanut butter, olive oil and erythritol in a small skillet over low heat without boiling for about 3 minutes. Remove from heat. In a bowl, beat egg yolks until creamy.

Ingredients:

- ✓ 1 tbsp olive oil
- ✓ 2 egg yolks
- ✓ ½ cup pecans, chopped

- ❖ Stir the eggs into the cream mixture. Continue stirring until a thick batter has formed, about 3 minutes. Pour the cream mixture into a bowl. Place in the refrigerator for 30 minutes. Stir in confectioners' sweetener.
- ❖ Pour mixture into ice cream maker and churn according to manufacturer's instructions. Stir in pecan later and spoon mixture into baking dish. Freeze for 2 hours before serving.

Nutrition: Kcal 302, Fat 32g, Net Carbs 2g, Protein 5g

121)   Coffee Fat Bombs

Preparation Time: 3 minutes + cooling time

Servings: 6

Ingredients:

- ✓ 6 tbsp prepared coffee at room temperature
- ✓ 1 ½ cups mascarpone cheese
- ✓ ½ cup melted butter

Ingredients:

- ✓ 3 tbsp unsweetened cocoa powder
- ✓ ¼ cup erythritol

Directions:

- ❖ Beat mascarpone, butter, cocoa powder, erythritol and coffee with a hand mixer until creamy and fluffy, about 1 minute.

- ❖ Fill muffin pans and freeze for 3 hours until firm.

Nutrition: Kcal 145, fat 14g, net carbs 2g, protein 4g

122)   Mixed Berry and Mascarpone Bowl

Preparation Time: 8 minutes

Servings: 4

Ingredients:

- ✓ 4 cups of Greek yogurt
- ✓ Liquid stevia to taste
- ✓ 1 ½ cups mascarpone cheese

Ingredients:

- ✓ 1 ½ cups blueberries and raspberries
- ✓ 1 cup toasted pecans

Directions:

- ❖ Mix the yogurt, stevia and mascarpone in a bowl until evenly combined.

- ❖ Divide the mixture among 4 bowls, divide the berries and pecans on top of the cream. Serve the dessert immediately.

Nutrition: Kcal 480, Fat 40g, Net Carbs 5g, Protein 20g

123)   Crazy Delicious Pudding

Preparation Time: 45 minutes

Servings: 2

Ingredients:

- ✓ 1 tangerine, sliced
- ✓ Juice of 2 tangerines
- ✓ 3 tbsp stevia
- ✓ 4 ounces of melted ghee
- ✓ ½ cup water

Ingredients:

- ✓ 2 tbsp flax meal
- ✓ ¾ cup coconut flour
- ✓ 1 tsp baking powder
- ✓ ¾ cup almonds, ground
- ✓ Olive oil cooking spray
- ❖ Add the water to the Instant Pot, place the trivet on top, add the pan, cover and cook on high heat for 35 minutes.
- ❖ Set aside to cool, slice and serve.
- ❖ Enjoy!

Directions:

- ❖ Grease a baking dish, arrange sliced tangerine on the bottom and set aside.
- ❖ In a bowl, mix ghee with stevia, flax meal, almonds, tangerine juice, flour and baking powder, stir and spread over tangerine slices.

Nutrition: Calories 200 | Fat: 2g | Carbohydrates: 3g | Protein: 4g | Fiber: 2g | Sugar: 0g

THE PALEO DIET FOR MEN: The Guide with 150+ Grain- and Gluten-Free Recipes to Lose Weight and Start Whole-Foods Lifestyle!

CONCLUSIONS

The Paleo diet is a lifestyle answer that is steadily gaining popularity these days. Many people are finding this diet very beneficial to their health. It is a natural diet that focuses on whole and unprocessed foods.

With the Paleo diet, you can lose weight and feel healthier. The Paleo diet is low in sugar. It is free of grains, dairy, legumes, refined carbohydrates, and processed foods. This means you will eat natural foods rich in vitamins, minerals, antioxidants, and fiber.

The Paleo diet helps in the prevention of various diseases. Some benefits of the Paleo diet include an improved immune system and a reduced chance of developing cancer and heart disease. The Paleo diet is a way of eating that became popular in the early 2000s. It is a lifestyle that hunter-gatherers practiced for millions of years before agriculture. One of the key ideas is that we have evolved to eat foods that are in season. It's a way to ensure we get nutrients from our food. A simple way to implement this way of eating is to find whole, fresh foods in season. The Paleo diet does not encourage processed foods, fast foods, or refined sugars or oils. It is considered ideal for keeping the mind and body healthy. It encourages the consumption of fresh foods and minimizes exposure to chemicals such as preservatives and artificial additives. The Paleo diet is a way of life for Paleolithic humans. This means that the way they ate differed from the way we eat today. This diet is designed to mimic the eating habits of our ancestors. The Paleo diet focuses on eating foods that are rich in vitamins and minerals. These foods include fish, meat, vegetables, fruits, nuts, and seeds. This diet also encourages low glycaemic index fruits and vegetables.

As beneficial as this diet can be to your health, it also has drawbacks. For example, individuals who follow the Paleo diet may suffer from nutrient deficiencies. This type of diet can also lead to a higher incidence of health problems such as acne and cancer.

However, you address these issues, you need to know what the Paleo diet is and how it is used today.

9 781802 748048